The Divorce Process: A Handbook for Clinicians

The Divorce Process: A Handbook for Clinicians

Craig A. Everett
Editor

The Haworth Press
New York • London

The Divorce Process: A Handbook for Clinicians has also been published as *Journal of Divorce*, Volume 10, Numbers 1/2, Fall/Winter 1986.

The Haworth Press, 12 West 32 Street, New York, NY 10001
EUROSPAN/Haworth, 3 Henrietta Street, London WC2E 8LU England

Library of Congress Cataloging-in-Publication Data

The Divorce process.

Published also as v. 10, no. 1-2 of the Journal of divorce.
1. Divorce therapy. 2. Divorce – Psychological aspects. 3. Children of divorced parents – Mental health. I. Everett, Craig A.
RC488.6.D57 1987 616.89 87-8513
ISBN 0-86656-662-7

The Divorce Process: A Handbook for Clinicians

Journal of Divorce
Volume 10, Numbers 1/2

CONTENTS

Introduction

The well-documented rate of divorce and family dissolution has spawned a broad range of investigations over the past two decades. For the most part, the resulting literature on the experience of divorce has examined both etiological and subsequent adjustment variables ranging from demography and economics to role conflict, grief and reorganization. By far the greatest portion of the literature has focused on the vulnerabilities of parent-child adjustments. All of this literature has provided a substantially comprehensive and empirically grounded body of knowledge.

However, in the real world, it is the practitioners—the clinicians, the attorneys and judges, and the mediators—who must struggle in a face to face relationship with the anger and pain of parting spouses and disrupted childhoods. Unfortunately, neither the divorce field nor the clinical disciplines themselves have yet evolved clear or definitive models of clinical assessment or intervention to aid the therapists in working with divorcing families. It is particularly noteworthy that the family therapy field, which has made such great strides in theory and practice over the past decade, has not effectively addressed the needs of this area of clinical practice.

This work is an effort to blend a variety of contributions—both descriptive, theoretical, and empirical—into a single volume which focuses a variety of resources for the clinician. The reader will not find consistent theoretical threads or congruent clinical models, but rather a rich variety of clinically useful materials from which to pick and choose. The works are organized along a general continuum from background theory to marital interaction to the definition of clinical dysfunctions in children of divorce to specific clinical features of childhood developmental levels to post-divorce reorganization and finally to models of group work.

Throughout there has been an effort to create an interplay between theoretical propositions, empirical data and clinical models. It is perhaps a misnomer, or at least premature, to describe such a work as a "handbook," but it is intended as a start in defining the field and represents the best that is available.

Craig A. Everett, PhD
Editor

The Divorce Process: A Handbook for Clinicians

BACKGROUND

The Developmental Course of Conflict in the Marital Dissolution Process

James J. Ponzetti, Jr.
Rodney M. Cate

ABSTRACT. The purpose of this study was to examine the developmental trend of conflict from the initial recognition that the marriage may dissolve to its legal termination. One hundred and seven participants completed a retrospective interview concerning their divorces. Levels of conflict, trust, ambivalence, love, and maintenance were assessed across three time periods during the divorce process. Conflict increased significantly from initial recognition to discussion and decreased significantly once action to secure a legal dissolution was initiated. The strongest predictors of conflict during the marital dissolution process were trust, ambivalence, and maintenance behaviors. Discussion focuses on the changing role of conflict during the divorce process.

Conflict is an inevitable component of, if not endemic to, marriage and family relationships (Sprey, 1979). In fact, the negotiation of conflict may be one of the primary means partners use to determine the viability of their relationships (Kelley, 1979; Scanzoni, 1972). Recent studies of marital interaction have uncovered consistent differences between distressed and nondistressed couples in commu-

James J. Ponzetti, Jr., PhD, is Assistant Professor, Department of Family Studies, University of New Mexico, Albuquerque, NM 87131.

Rodney M. Cate, PhD, is Chairman and Professor, Department of Child and Family Studies, Washington State University, Pullman, WA 99164.

nication, problem-solving, and conflict. There is considerable evidence, as Glick and Gross (1975) have maintained, that the process of interaction during conflict is a critical determinant of marital satisfaction. The couple's ability to reach agreement and resolve relationship problems may be the critical resource contributing to marital quality, and thereby to marital stability (Gottman, 1979; Lewis & Spanier, 1979). Some researchers consider the inability of one partner to change the other's behavior in a desired direction, as the crucial factor in the breakdown, and possible dissolution, of marital relationships (Patterson & Hops, 1972; Patterson, Hops, & Weiss, 1975).

Peterson (1983) has defined conflict as the interpersonal process that takes place whenever the actions of one partner interfere with the actions of the other partner. Since divorce is rarely a mutually agreed upon course of action (Kressel, Jaffee, Tuchman, Watson, & Deutsch, 1980; Vaughan, 1979; Wallerstein & Kelly, 1980), the process of marital dissolution is often conflictive, in that the decision of one spouse to terminate the marriage may interfere with the other spouse's wish to maintain the relationship. Although the developmental course of conflict has been studied as couples move toward marriage (Braiker & Kelley, 1979) and as premarital relationships develop and dissolve (Lloyd & Cate, 1985), its course has yet to be considered during marital dissolution.

THE PROCESS OF MARITAL DISSOLUTION

Marital dissolution involves the social, emotional, and legal process through which former spouses move from marriage to another lifestyle; that is to say, divorce is not a single event that occurs at one point in time (Baxter & Philpott, 1980; Kitson, Babri, & Roach, 1985; Duck, 1982). Yet, a considerable amount of research has focused on the adjustment to marital termination as if implying that the legal decree is the single most important event during the dissolution process. Surprisingly little is known about what takes place between marital partners as they move toward this event (Kressel et al., 1980). Therefore, this study will focus on the spouses' perceptions of their interaction before the legal divorce decree was secured.

STAGES OF DIVORCE

Researchers have conceptualized various stages of the marital dissolution process (Lyon, Silverman, Howe, Bishop, & Armstrong, 1985; Price-Bonham, Wright, & Pittman 1983; Salts, 1979). These various models can be approximated by four sequential time periods: recognition, discussion, action, and postdissolution.

Recognition. The recognition process begins when either partner becomes cognizant of significant problems, dissatisfaction, or discontent such that the stability of the marriage is called into question. Recognition is essentially an intrapersonal and cognitive period (Duck, 1982). The recognition of discontent usually follows a period of marital stress in which tensions within the couple remain covert (Brown, 1976; Vaughan, 1979; Lee, 1984). Marital stress may occur whenever the marital expectations of either spouse are not realized. Unmet expectations may lead to a conflicted marriage as couples perceive a growing distance between them. This in turn leads to serious communication problems and regressive cycles in which spouses recycle resentment, silence, lack of self-disclosure, and avoidance of serious issues (Bradford, 1980). Marriages may continue in this fashion for years before unrealized dreams, unattained goals, and unfulfilled expectations create further resentments, bitterness, and boredom.

Discussion. The discussion time period begins when the intrapersonal recognition of dissatisfaction is shared with others, such as the spouse, a counselor, lover, or friend. This discussion is characterized by more than simply conversation. It is of a more serious nature. The dissatisfied spouse is in the process of redefining the relationship in light of the discontent that became evident during the preceding period (Vaughan, 1979). The period is marked by attempts at reconciliation, a decline in feelings of love and intimacy, and finally a break in the public facade of solidarity (Kressel & Deutsch, 1977).

The first indication that either spouse is ready to begin restructuring their lives is their willingness to accept their role in the divorce decision and its outcomes (Newman & Langer, 1981). When the individual is unable to do this, often indicated by continuing anger toward the spouse or by blaming the spouse for the marital problems, there remains considerable emotional involvement with the spouse. Conflict is not an uncommon manifestation of this period. In fact, either spouse may utilize conflict as a means of maintaining the relationship if they are unwilling or unready to begin restructuring their own lives (Brown, 1976).

Lyon et al. (1985) noted that this decision-making phase is characterized by increased conflict, ambivalence, and emotional upheaval. Vaughan (1979) also noted that heightened uncertainty is evident during this time, especially if a new definition of the couple's identity cannot be reached. The ambiguity surrounding the relationship hinders the reorganization of the marital system.

Furthermore, although many researchers view this discussion as taking place only between the marital partners (Vaughan, 1979; Duck, 1982; Lee, 1984), it is not unlikely that discussion may occur between the dissatisfied spouse and someone other than the partner. For instance, the dissatisfied partner may discuss his or her discontent with a lover or friend and, only later, inform the spouse of the decision to divorce without providing an opportunity for the spouse to negotiate the future of the marriage at all.

Action. The third period occurs once either spouse initiates any action to secure a legal dissolution. The legal formalization of divorce, the economic settlement concerning division of shared assets, arrangements for child care and fulfillment of parental obligations, and possible community disapproval all come into play as those divorcing share their marital plight with family, friends, and the greater community. Intense feelings of ambivalence about ending the marriage continue. Oftentimes anxiety over separation and a brief renewal of intimacy manifests itself at this time (Kressel & Deutsch, 1977; Vaughan, 1979; Weiss, 1976). Yet, as tensions are exacerbated, conflict and resentments develop which continue to break threads of trust, respect, and mutual attraction. This period is commonly quite difficult (Albrecht, 1980; Lyon et al., 1985).

Postdissolution. The postdissolution period begins once the partners accept the inevitability that the marriage will end. This period involves reflection upon the reasons for the divorce and the creation of an acceptable personal account regarding the dissolved marital relationship (Duck, 1982). Former partners must also make arrangements for dealing with the "continuities" which continue to exist in spite of the divorce (Vaughan, 1979). For instance, relationships with former in-laws or couple friends may be continued. This postdissolution period has received considerable attention, but there remains a paucity of research which focuses on the predivorce periods (Kitson et al., 1985).

SALIENT DIMENSIONS DURING DISSOLUTION

Empirical investigations have just begun to consider how salient relationship dynamics change over the course of the dissolution process. Kressel et al. (1980) considered the degree of conflict and ambivalence as crucial factors in differentiating how well couples adjusted to divorce. Unfortunately, this research can only be suggestive of what takes place between spouses as they move toward divorce because it is based only on the experiences of a small purposive sample of 14 couples. Hagestad and Smyer (1982) distinguished between orderly and disorderly divorces on the basis that, in the former, spouses had gone through a psychological divorce before the legal one. Psychological divorce involves the spouse coming to terms with the breakdown of trust, resolving ambivalent feelings, disconnecting their identity from marital roles, and withdrawal of feelings of love and emotional investment in each other (Bohannon, 1970).

The postulation of stages of divorce offers a useful conceptualizaton of the experience of dissolving marital relationships. However, further research is needed to clarify how relationship dynamics change as individuals dissolve their marriages. Past research has identified the salience of conflict, ambivalence, trust, love, and maintenance behaviors (i.e., problem-solving and self-disclosure) in explicating the divorce process. Therefore, the purpose of this paper will be twofold. First, it will examine the developmental trend of conflict from the initial recognition that the marriage may dissolve to its legal termination. Second, the interrelationships of conflict with trust, ambivalence, love, and maintenance behaviors will be investigated through three time periods during the divorce process.

METHOD

Participants

This study is based on interviews and questionnaires completed by 107 divorced individuals (57 men and 50 women). The participants were predominantly white, Protestant, had a mean age of 36.7 years, and had been married for an average of 10.2 years and separated an average of 43.8 months before their divorce. At the time of the interview, they had been legally divorced for an average of 32.9

months. Most participants had attended some college (43.0%), with a considerable number completing college (25.2%) or graduate and professional school (23.4%). Approximately 75% were employed at the time of the study primarily in professional (18.7%), semi-professional (22.4%), or skilled (24.3%) occupations.

Two methods were employed to promote a good response rate. First, the population of men and women who were either petitioners, copetitioners, or respondents in petitions for dissolution of marriage, filed in Benton County, Oregon within the preceding 18 months were obtained from county records. A letter was sent to possible participants explaining the research project and asking for their cooperation.

The second method of recruiting took place concurrently with the first and was intended to incorporate potential participants who were not, for whatever reasons, reached via local courthouse records. Local singles organizations, such as Parents Without Partners, were contacted for possible participants. The only restriction on sample inclusion was that the final divorce must have been granted. As volunteers agreed to participate, an interview was scheduled.

Procedure

This study utilized a retrospective interview technique, because it provides an acceptable methodology for mapping the developmental process of relationships (Huston, Surra, Fitzgerald, & Cate, 1981; Lloyd & Cate, 1985). This technique provided a means by which to outline, within a specific time and behavioral frame, the marital dissolution process.

Data were gathered through a two-hour personal interview, and paper and pencil questionnaires. The interview was comprised of two parts. First, participants were asked to trace, retrospectively, the changes in the perceived probability of divorce from the point when significant dissatisfaction with the marriage was initially recognized until the date of the final divorce decree. The changes were plotted on a "chance of divorce" graph. This graph became a pictorial representation of the divorce process over time. The participants were then asked to indicate the portion of the graph during which: (a) they recognized significant marital dissatisfaction on their part or that of their spouse that made them think their problems might lead to divorce (intrapersonal recognition), (b) they openly discussed with other people the possibility that their marriage might end in divorce (interpersonal discussion), and (c) either partner initiated action toward securing a legal divorce decree. Once these periods were identified, they were marked on the graph providing the participants a clear event-oriented picture of when these three periods had occurred in the dissolution process.

The next portion of the interview consisted of assessing the levels of love, conflict, maintenance, ambivalence, and trust in the marital relationship as the couple moved towards divorce. Participants completed three questionnaires which corresponded to the three time periods outlined on the graph. Each questionnaire contained scales that measured the amount of conflict, love, maintenance, ambivalence, and trust during that particular period.

Throughout the analyses, attention was paid to potential differences between men and women in their retrospective accounts about their marriages. Research concerning sex differences in reaction to divorce are not conclusive. Weiss (1975) noted that marital separation is as distressing for men as for women. However, Bloom and Caldwell (1981) and Albrecht (1980) found differences in adjustment at different periods during the divorce process.

Measures

The dimensions of conflict, ambivalence, maintenance, and love were assessed with the scales developed by Braiker and Kelley (1979). Conflict was measured by the five items that assessed the amount of overt conflict, arguments, and communication of negative affect in the marital relationship. For example, ''How often did you feel angry or resentful toward your spouse?'' Ambivalence was assessed by five items that tapped feelings of uncertainty, confusion, and anxiety concerning commitment to the partner. For example, ''How ambivalent or unsure were you about continuing in the relationship with your spouse?'' Maintenance was assessed by five items that tapped both the communication of feelings and needs to one's partner and discussions directed at solving relationship problems. For example, ''To what extent did you try to change your behavior to help solve certain problems between you and your spouse?'' Love was assessed by ten items that measured feelings of closeness, belonging and commitment. For example, ''How close did you feel to your spouse?'' Participants were asked to indicate the degree to which each feeling was true of their relationship on a nine-point Likert scale of 1 (not true at all) to 9 (very true).

Trust was measured with the dyadic trust scale developed by Larzelere and Huston (1980). This scale assessed the extent that a person believes another person to be benevolent and honest. The scale consisted of eight items, each measured on a seven-point Likert scale.

RESULTS AND DISCUSSION

Developmental Trends

A repeated measures analysis of variance was performed to analyze the developmental trend of conflict. This analysis checked for significant differences in conflict between gender, who initiated the divorce process and time periods. Results indicated that the developmental trend of conflict was significant over time, $F\ (2,186) = 14.86$, $p < .0001$. Post-hoc analysis (Scheffe, $p < .05$) revealed that conflict increased significantly from recognition to discussion and decreased significantly from discussion to action. No other significant main effects or interactions were found.

These findings support the idea that as individuals move toward the legal termination of their marriage, the level of conflict changes. Early in the dissolution process the realization, on the part of either spouse, of significant dissatisfaction that may lead to divorce is usually intrapersonal; that is, not shared with anyone else. Once either partner shares their concerns with someone else and some form of discussion concerning the nature or future course of their relationship begins, conflict between spouses increases. The reconstruction of the marital relationship in light of discontent on the part of either spouse may clarify differing expectations or decisions concerning the stability of the marriage. This uncertainty may explain the increase in conflict. Levels of conflict reach their peak during this discussion phase and then decrease after action is taken to secure a legal decree of dissolution. Perhaps the relatively high levels of interpersonal conflict seen during the discussion phase was indicative of a "last ditch" effort to salvage an already deteriorating marriage.

The Role of Conflict

The means of love, ambivalence, maintenance, conflict, and trust for each time period reveal that these dimensions do evidence significant change during the dissolution process (see Table 1). Ambivalence and conflict increased during the discussion period and subsequently decreased once action was taken to terminate the marriage. Trust, love, and maintenance behaviors decreased throughout the divorce process.

The second purpose of this study was to examine how love, maintenance, ambivalence, and trust interrelate with conflict at three time periods during the process of marital dissolution. Multiple regression analyses were performed for each time period with conflict as the dependent measure. The independent variables included in these analyses were love, maintenance, ambivalence, trust, gender, and four interaction terms. Each interaction term represented gender, which was coded as an indicator variable, multiplied by each of the independent variables. Since no significant interactions were found, only the main effects are discussed.

Results indicated that the regression equation was significant during each time priod: recognition, F (5, 101) = 6.79, p < .001; discussion, F (5,96) = 11.07, p < .001; action, F (9,96) = 8.73, p < .001. Multiple R values ranged as follows: recognition, R = .502; discussion, R = .605; and action, R = .448.

In order to compare across the regressions for each time period, the unstandardized Betas for each equation are presented in Table 2. Only the dimensions of ambivalence, trust, and maintenance changed significantly in relation to conflict as spouses moved from intrapersonal recognition to securing the dissolution of their marriage.

Love was not significantly related to conflict (given that ambivalence, trust, maintenance, and gender were already in the model and thus controlled for) during the dissolution process. This finding was not expected. Weiss (1975) has noted that the loss of love and attachment due to divorce produces intense feelings of distress and discomfort, and subsequent feelings of anger are typical. Spanier

Table 1: Means on Relationship Dimensions

Dimension	Time Period		
	Recognition	Discussion	Action
Conflict	27.48	30.01	23.79
Ambivalence	23.79	25.05	16.56
Love	60.45	50.23	33.06
Maintenance	25.50	24.64	14.69
Trust	27.39	24.61	21.73

Table 2: Unstandardized Regression Coefficients for Independent Variables Regressed on Conflict at Each of Three Time Periods

	Recognition	Discussion	Action
Ambivalence	0.2540**	0.3569***	0.3696***
Maintenance	0.3421***	0.1648	0.2448*
Love	-0.0039	0.0040	0.0453
Trust	-0.1303*	-0.2637***	-0.3587***
Gender	-0.5771	-0.1451	0.1001
Constant	16.4477	23.2948	20.3799
Multiple R	0.5015	0.6048	0.6692

* p .05. ** p .004. *** p .001

and Thompson (1984) report that such anger encourages interpersonal conflict between spouses. One possible explanation for the lack of any significant relationship between love and conflict may be that by the time either partner recognized marital dissatisfaction such that dissolution was considered the remedy the external factors involved in divorce, such as division of assets, may be more important in explaining the degree of conflict than affective issues such as love. Love did decrease as individuals moved closer to securing a divorce; however, it appears that there are more salient dimensions, such as trust and ambivalence, which offer better explanations of marital conflict as the relationship dissolves.

Because marital partners remain attached to each other and are simultaneously angry with each other, the relationship of divorcing spouses is intensely ambivalent (Weiss, 1975). Ambivalence was significantly positively related to conflict during the divorce process. As interpersonal conflict increased, ambivalence similarly increased. It is not clear from these data whether an increase in conflict leads to an increase in ambivalence or whether ambivalence promotes conflict. It is likely a reciprocal relationship. No matter how committed the individual appears to a particular course of action, there is apt to be intense ambivalence regarding the spouse. Weiss (1975) and Kressel et al. (1980) report that the management of ambivalent feelings regarding the break-up is one of the most prominent problems spouses must deal with during the divorce process.

Trust was significantly negatively related to conflict during all three time periods. As conflict increased during the process, dyadic trust decreased. Bohannon (1970) noted that the breakdown of trust was a typical characteristic of the psychological divorce. The presence of conflict during the process of marital dissolution may emphasize the waning commitment between spouses toward their relationship. Larzelere and Huston (1980) proposed that dyadic trust seems to be a prerequisite for commitment. These findings offer some support for a reciprocal relationship in that the divorcing spouse's renegotiation of their commitment to their marriage may promote conflict and as conflict increases, dyadic trust decreases.

Maintenance behaviors also changed in their relationship to conflict over the course of the dissolution. Maintenance behaviors, such as self-disclosure and problem-solving, were significantly positively related to conflict during the recognition and action time periods. Levinger (1976) has hypothesized that in long-term relationships, such as marriage, as either partner recognizes the possibility of divorce, the salience of the costs and benefits of the relationship begin to receive more attention. Since maintenance includes primarily communication behaviors between partners aimed at reducing the cost and maximizing the benefits from the relationship, it is not too surprising to find that spouses attend to such behaviors once they recognize that the future of their relationship is in jeopardy. In fact, such recognition may promote these behaviors in an attempt to retrieve an already troubled marriage. However, it seems that even during this initial period of the divorce process, the more one partner spends time disclosing to their spouse and trying to work out problems, the more arguments, anger, and resentment increase. These results may be due to the presence of regressive cycles in which, spouses recycle resentment, lack of self-disclosure, and avoidance behavior as they ponder the future course of the marriage (Bradford, 1980). Maintenance behaviors were not related to conflict when either spouse was actively questioning and discussing the viability of their marriage with others. Ambivalence and trust were the only significant predictors of conflict during this discussion period. This may be explained in that once either spouse initiates discussions with others concerning the possibility of divorce their psychological resources may be directed away from further efforts to maintain what they perceive as a troubled marriage. Or perhaps, during this discussion period, people simply see conflict and maintenance behaviors as serving different purposes within the marital relationship.

Divorcing spouses are often angry with each other not only because of genuine conflicts of interest but because they blame each other for their distress. Conflicts sometimes appear to be used as a means of keeping the relationship alive through transfusions of hostility. Yet, maintenance during the action period probably has less to do with maintaining a terminal relationship than it does with problems that must be resolved to secure legal dissolution. The adversarial nature of the courts, and the antagonism between partners which it fosters, does not promote effective problem-solving, but rather encourages conflict. Quarrels are likely to occur in relation to property, money, and custody if children are present. Thus, although problem-solving behaviors increase once action is initiated, so does conflict between the couple, and attorneys and the courts may be needed to assist them in resolving problematic issues.

CONCLUSION

This study has examined the role of conflict during the dissolution of marital relationships. Dyadic trust, ambivalence, and maintenance were found to be significant predictors of the level of conflict as marital relationships moved toward dissolution. The level of conflict was negatively related to trust and positively related to ambivalence and maintenance. Thus, the presence of high levels of conflict during the dissolution process reflected low levels of dyadic trust and high levels of ambivalence and maintenance behaviors. It appears that early in the process spouses were attempting to negotiate the viability of their marriage both through conflict and maintenance behaviors such as talking things out. Yet, as spouses began to discuss the possibility of ending their marriage with others, levels of conflict reflected greater feelings of ambivalence toward the relationship. Maintenance behaviors were no longer significant predictors during this time. This finding appears to support Bradford's (1980) contention that as a marriage deteriorates the partners focus their time and energy on things outside the relationship itself. In addition, dyadic trust decreased throughout the process of divorce. This, too, may partially account for the spouses' unwillingness to work together in order to resolve their concerns and maintain their marriage. Although love was found to be a salient dimension in predicting conflict during the dissolution of premarital relationships (Lloyd & Cate, 1985), it was not found to be so during marital dissolution. One explanation offered for this was that feelings of love may become relatively less important by the time either spouse opts for dissolving the marital relationship.

These findings have implications both for service delivery aimed at assisting couples who are dissolving their marriages and for future research. The data suggest that counselors and other professionals working with troubled marriages should be sensitive to the many changes which accompany the process of marital dissolution. Moreover, the efficacy of any intervention with divorcing couples may be related to the time during the process that such intervention is sought. Since conflict has been shown to differentiate distressed and nondistressed couples, it follows that the reduction of conflict may enable spouses to consider other relationship concerns. This research found the strongest predictors of conflict during the dissolution process were the level of trust between spouses, the ambivalence they feel toward their marriage, and the behaviors they engage in to solve problems and maintain their relationship. Thus, counselors may intervene to build dyadic trust, decrease feelings of ambivalence, or teach effective problem-solving in an attempt to manage marital conflict which may arise due to the situation.

Although certain limitations accompany any methodology, retrospective interviews have been effectively employed in several recent studies of premarital and marital relationships (Lloyd & Cate, 1985; Kelly, Huston, & Cate, 1985; Surra, 1985). Retrospective interviews provide not only valuable descriptive data that can direct future research concerning the development of close relationships but are also particularly useful for gathering information about the dissolution process (Kitson et al., 1985). Levinger (1983) has pointed out that distance from the marriage allows former partners to discern what occurred within the relationship without being hindered by the emotional involvement and upheaval that oftentimes complicates the process. Many researchers have emphasized that it takes several years to adjust to the divorce experience (Lyon et al., 1985; Weiss, 1975). Therefore, retrospective information about marital dissolution is probably more accurate than data collected during the divorce. Much more work remains to be done concerning what occurs before the final divorce decree is granted. The findings presented here offer a beginning.

BIBLIOGRAPHY

Albrecht, S.L. (1980) Reactions and Adjustment to Divorce: Differences in the Experiences of Males and Females. *Family Relations, 29,* 59–68.

Baxter, L. & Philpott, J. (1980) Relationship Disengagement: A Process View. Paper presented at the Speech Communication Association convention, November.

Bloom, B. and Caldwell, R.A. (1981) Sex differences in Adjustment During the Process of Marital Separation. *Journal of Marriage and the Family, 43* (3), 693–701.

Bradford, L. (1980) The Death of a Dyad. In B.W. Morse & L.A. Phelps (Eds.) *Interpersonal Communication: A Relational Perspective.* Minneapolis, MN: Burgess Publishing Co.

Braiker, H.B. & Kelley, H.H. (1979) Conflict in the development of Close Relationships. In R. Burgess & T. Huston (Eds.), *Social Exchange in Developing Relationships.* New York: Academic Press.

Brown, E.M. (1976) A Model of the Divorce Process. *Conciliation Courts Review, 14,* 1–11.

Duck, S. (1982) A Typology of Relationship Disengagement and Dissolution. In S. Duck (Ed.) *Personal Relationships 4. Dissolving Personal Relationships.* London: Academic Press.

Glick, B. and Gross, S.J. (1975) Marital Interaction and Marital Conflict: A Critical Evaluation of Current Research Strategies. *Journal of Marriage and the Family, 37* (3), 505–514.

Gottman, J.M. (1979) *Marital Interaction: Experimental Investigations.* New York: Academic Press.

Hagestad, G. & Smyer, M. (1982) Dissolving Long Term Relationships: Patterns of Divorcing in Middle Age. In S. Duck (Ed.) *Personal Relationships 4. Dissolving Personal Relationships.* London Academic Press.

Kelley, H.H. (1979) *Personal Relationships: Their Structure and Processes.* Hillsdale, N.J.: Lawrence Erlbaum Associates.

Kelly, C., Huston, T., & Cate, R. (1985) Premarital Relationship Correlates of the Erosion of Satisfaction in Marriage. *Journal of Social and Personal Relationships, 2* (2), 167–178.

Kitson, G., Babri, K.B., & Roach, M. (1985) Who Divorces and Why: A Review. *Journal of Family Issues, 6* (3), 253–294.

Kressel, K. & Deutsch, M. (1979) Divorce Therapy. An In-Depth Survey of Therapists' Views. *Family Process, 16* (4), 413–444.

Kressel, K., Jaffee, N., Tuchman, B., Watson, C., & Deutsch, M. (1980) A Typology of Divorcing Couples: Implications for Mediation and the Divorce Process. *Family Process, 19* (2), 101–116.

Larzelere, R.E. & Huston, T.L. (1980) The Dyadic Trust Scale: Toward Understanding Interpersonal Trust in Close Relationships. *Journal of Marriage and the Family, 42* (3), 595–604.

Lee, L. (1984) Sequences in Separation: A Framework for Investigating Endings of the Personal (Romantic) Relationship. *Journal of Social and Personal Relationships, 1* (1), 49–74.

Levinger, G. (1976) A Social Psychological Perspective on Marital Dissolution. *Journal of Social Issues, 32* (1), 21–47.

Levinger, G. (1983) Development and Change. In H. Kelley, E. Berscheid, A. Christensen, J. Harvey, T. Huston, G. Levinger, E. McClintock, L. Peplau, & D. Peterson (Eds.) *Close Relationships.* New York: W.H. Freeman & Company.

Lewis, R.A. & Spanier, G.B. (1979) Theorizing About the Quality and Stability of Marriage. In W.R. Burr, R. Hill, F.I. Nye, I.L. Reiss (Eds.) *Contemporary Theories About the Family, v.1,* New York: The Free Press.

Lloyd, S.A. and Cate, R.M. (1985) The Developmental Course of Conflict in Premarital Relationship Dissolution. *Journal of Personal and Social Relationships, 2* (2), 179–194.

Lyon, E., Silverman, M., Howe, G., Bishop, G., & Armstrong, B. (1985) Stages of Divorce: Implications for Service Delivery. *Social Casework, 66* (5), 259–267.

Newman, H.M. and Langer, E.J. (1981) Post-Divorce Adaptation and the Attribution of Responsibility. *Sex Roles, 7* (3), 223–232.

Noller, P. (1984) *Nonverbal Communication and Marital Interaction.* Elmsford, N.Y.: Pergamon Press, Inc.

Patterson, G.D. & Hops, H. (1972) Coercion, A game for two: Intervention techniques for Marital Conflict. In R.E. Ulrich & P. Mountjoy (Eds.) *The Experimental Analysis of Social Behavior.* New York: Appleton-Century-Crofts.

Patterson, G.D., Hops, H., & Weiss, R.L. (1975) Interpersonal Skills Training for Couples in Early Stages of Conflict. *Journal of Marriage and the Family, 37,* 295–302.

Peterson, D.R. (1983) Conflict. In H. Kelley, E. Berscheid, A. Christensen, J. Harvey, T. Huston, G. Levinger, E. McClintock, L. Peplau, & D. Peterson (Eds.) *Close Relationships.* New York: W.H. Freeman & Company.

Price-Bonham, S., Wright, D., & Pittman, J. (1983) Divorce: A Frequent "Alternative" in the 1970's. In E. Macklin & R. Rubin (Eds.) *Contemporary Families and Alternative Lifestyles.* Beverly Hills: Sage Publications.

Salts, C. (1979) Divorce Process: Integration of Theory. *Journal of Divorce, 2* (3), 253–240.

Scanzoni, J. (1972) *Sexual Bargaining: Power Politics in American Marriage.* Englewood Cliffs, N.J.: Prentice-Hall.

Spanier, G.B. & Thompson, L. (1974) *Parting: The Aftermath of Separation and Divorce.* Beverly Hills, CA: Sage Publications.

Sprey, J. (1979) Conflict Theory and the Study of Marriage and the Family. In W. R. Burr, R.H. N, F.I. Nye & I.L. Reiss (Eds.) *Contemporary Theories About the Family, v.2.* New York: The Free Press.

Surra, C. (1985) Courtship Types: Variations in Interdependence Between Partners and Social Networks. *Journal of Personality and Social Psychology, 49* (2), 357–375.

Vaughan, D. (1979) Uncoupling: The Process of Moving From One Lifestyle to Another. *Alternative Lifestyles, 2* (4), 415–442.

Wallerstein, J.S. & Kelly, J.B. (1980) *Surviving the Break-up: How Children and Parents Cope with Divorce.* New York: Basic Books.

Weiss, R.S. (1975) *Marital Separation.* New York: Basic Books.

Weiss, R.S. (1976) The Emotional Impact of Marital Separation. *Journal of Social Issues, 32* (1), 135–145.

The Grief Resolution Process in Divorce: Phase II

John F. Crosby
Sandra K. Lybarger
Richard L. Mason

ABSTRACT. Building on a pilot study published in the *Journal of Divorce* (Fall, 1983), the work reported in phase two is based on 141 responses to a questionnaire rather than personal first-person essay accounts employed in phase one. The model is a $3 \times 3 \times 3$ taxonomy: three process stages; three filing categories (Actives-Passives-Mutuals); and three variables (Affect-Cognition-Behavior). Utilizing clusters, (a semantic and perceptual representation of related emotions, thoughts, and behaviors by incorporating related words under a banner word representing the entire range) the results of phase two revealed twenty-five out of twenty-seven significant chi squares, indicating the modal frequency of responses at various stages in the divorce process. The recovery "lag" between actives and passives was not confirmed as in the 1983 pilot. The passive "lag" exists only in the second stage but does not extend into the post-divorce stage. The recovery pattern between the actives and the mutuals bears strong similarity, wherein the passive pattern in the first two stages is quite different.

This study is a continuation and revision of the study first reported in the *Journal of Divorce* (1983: Crosby, Gage and Raymond). The hypothesis of the original study remained essentially unchanged in the second phase: Persons who have experienced divorce will display a sequence of feelings, cognitions, and behaviors which progress in general sequence from denial to anger to

---

John F. Crosby, PhD, is Professor of Family Studies, University of Kentucky. Sandra K. Lybarger is a doctoral candidate in Counseling Psychology, University of Kentucky. Richard L. Mason, PhD, is in private practice in Louisville, KY. Data for this project was collected between 1982 and early 1985.

bargaining to depression to acceptance. (The addition of the word "cognitions" is the only change.)

The first phase utilized a convenience sample of seventeen persons who told their own story in essay form. The respondents attempted to address a series of guideline questions: The resulting accounts were analyzed independently and separately. Beyond the limitations of self-report and self-selection, the use of first person essay accounts proved to be non-economical in that the assignment was either too demanding in terms of time and effort or too painful in terms of recall and description. We stated in the first article (1983; Crosby, Gage and Raymond): "Between twenty-five and thirty people indicated to the researchers their willingness to participate in the study but that they experienced too great a level of pain as they opened the door of their memories and began to write their story. These persons reported that to continue the writing would be too painful and/or depressing."

The second phase of the study retained the same procedures and methodology of the first study with the exception of the instrument. The second phase utilized a three part questionnaire: Part I includes sixteen demographic and personal background questions; Part II includes twenty-nine questions directly related to the divorce experience; Part III is a single question requiring the respondent to classify emotions, thoughts, and behaviors according to twenty related events common to the grief resolution process.

Between 1980 and 1985, after the above stated change in instrumentation, one hundred and fifty-five completed questionnaires were receiving. Of these, one hundred and forty-one were acceptable for inclusion in the data analysis. The data reported in this study, as with the original study, includes only those marriages which were classified as operationally dysfunctional or incompatible (in contrast to marriages characterized by one mate being severely mentally–emotionally disturbed and/or wherein one mate is oppressive–abusive.)

REVIEW OF LITERATURE: 1980 TO 1985

The literature reviewed in the Phase One study focused on eight theoretical models of the divorce process. Four of these models were based on the behavior/event dimension: Waller's (1938/1951) seven alienation crises and four stages of readjustment to the loss of the mate; Bohannan's (1970) six stations of emotional divorce; and Kressel and Deutsch's (1977) four periods of psychic divorce. The remaining four models were based on the affective dimension: Herman's (1974) use of Kubler-Ross' five stages of the grief process; Defazio and Kleinbort's (1975) three stages of marital dissolution; Wiseman's (1975) five stages of emotional crisis; and Kraus' (1979) use of Falek and Britton's five phases of coping. The review of these eight models of the process of grief resolution was presented within a three part time frame, i.e., from first serious thought about divorce to separation and/or filing; from separation and/or filing to final decree; and from final decree to penultimate closure.

Our review of the literature since 1980 has revealed an effort in understanding the dimensions of meaning and belongingness in divorce (Hancock, 1980), a social-exchange emphasis on decision making in divorce (Albrecht and Kunz, 1980) crisis intervention via the use of divorce workshops (Davidoff and Schiller, 1983, and Dasteel, 1982), a study of sex differences in initiation and adjustment to divorce (Zeiss, Zeiss, and Johnson, 1980), social network changes (Daniels-Mohring and Berger, 1984), the impact of divorce (Kolevzon and Gottleib, 1983), loneliness in divorce (Woodward, Zabel, and Decosta, 1980), change over time in personality characteristics of divorced women (Spivey and Scherman, 1980), and several studies which consider the more global issue of loss and grieving (Heikkinen, 1981; Davenport, 1981; and Frears and Schneider, 1981).

The relationship between divorce and suicide has been studied by Stack (1980), and also by Wasserman (1984). Stack noted that a one percent increase in divorce was associated with a .54 percent increase in the suicide rate. Wasserman's findings "substantiate the hypothesis that the process of divorce increases the probability that individuals will commit suicide" (Wasserman, 1984).

Among the studies which bear a more direct relation to the entire process of grief resolution based on a functional model over the various phases and stages are the following. Kaslow (1984) employs a therapeutic treatment model based on Bohannan's six stages of divorce. Using pre, during, and post stages, Kaslow lists forty-two specific feelings which are predominant at different points in the six Bohannan stations of divorce. Kaslow further lists thirty-two actions/tasks which are predominant at different points in the Bohannan stations. Kaslow does not attempt to posit a cognition or "thoughts" category in her taxonomy. Writing for the benefit of the intervenor/therapist, Kaslow describes the appropriate therapeutic intervention for the Bohannan stations. A comparison of Kaslow's work with Phase One of our efforts should yield a functional–therapeutic synthesis without much conceptual difficulty because of the similarity of the models.

Saul and Scherman (1984) used twelve groups in their study of the relationship of divorce grief to personal adjustment. The twelve groups included Remarried male 6–18 months following divorce, Remarried male 19–36 months, Remarried female with children 6–18 months, Remarried female with children 19–36 months, Remarried female without children 19–36 months, Single female with children 6–18 months, Single female without children 6–18 months, and Single female without children 19–36 months. Saul and Scherman reported no statistical significant difference in their measures of grief and adjustment.

The significance of the Saul and Scherman study is the lack of meaningful variation among the 114 subjects distributed among the twelve groups. This is not meant to suggest that further research will not come to different conclusions regarding grief and personal adjustment. It does suggest, however, that gender, the absence or presence of children, and elapsed time since divorce may not be nearly as important to final resolution as was previously believed. The key variable in adjustment may well yet prove to be the grief work itself, i.e., the process of mourning and actively dealing with one's own sense of loss. This is not to disparage the "Correlates of Recovery" such as economic stability, physical health, emotional health, experience with previous loss and/or previous divorce(s), familial presence, expectations imposed by both self and others, defense mechanisms, values, religious beliefs, and one's personal definition of the meaning of marriage and/or divorce.

Spanier and Thompson (1983) utilized 205 respondents in an attempt to determine the response to marital termination in terms of relief, distress, or no-change. Spanier and Thompson were working with the terminal stage of marriage i.e., the final months of the marriage leading up to separation. Relief, distress, and no change were measured as post separation relief. Spanier and Thompson state "it is evident that females are more likely to be found in the relief and distress groups, and men are more likely to be found in the no change category." Spanier and Thompson further note that "those who are not as highly educated and on the receiving end of the divorce suggestion are most likely to experience distress, rather than relief or stability, after marital separation.'' The factor of gender difference in the Spanier and Thompson study is not in keeping with the Saul and Scherman study (1984). Further, the Spanier and Thompson data lend support to the Phase One conclusion of our previous study in terms of the passive agents lagging behind the active agents. Spanier and Thompson, as noted above, state that distress is most likely to be the outcome among those who were on the receiving end of the divorce suggestion.

Brown, Felton, Whiteman, and Manela (1980) also studied distress following separation. The sample included 192 respondents in the process of marital dissolution. The chief purpose of this study was to determine the role that prior attachment plays in the experience of post separation distress. The authors conclude that ''attachment seems to be a useful concept whose value is increased by distinguishing it from the global distress experienced after marital separation. Although not a complete explanation for the anguish that accompanies marital separation, it plays a major role in the emotional upheaval of separation.'' Attachment was also the main concern of Kitson, who devised a scale for the measurement of continuing affectional bonds (Kitson, 1982). Kitson confirms the difference between the active and passive agents in terms of attachment, i.e., greater feelings of attachment prevailed on the part of the passive agent. Kitson concludes that the loss of a relationship and the inherent attachment within that relationship, even if the relationship has turned sour, can produce distress. Kitson, with Sussman, also studied complaints, demographic characteristics, and symptoms of distress in divorce (Kitson and Sussman, 1982).

Thompson and Spanier (1983) dealt with the final stage, acceptance. ''Acceptance is highest among those men with a mutually-decided divorce, lowest among the spouse-initiated divorced men, with the self-initiated divorced men falling in between.'' Among females, ''although the effect on acceptance of source of the initial suggestion falls short of significance, the pattern is in the predicted direction and matches that found among men.''

Bloom and Caldwell studied male-female differences in adjustment during the process of separation (1981). Preseparation women reported poorer psychological adjustment than preseparation men. Early postseparation men reported ''substantially poorer adjustment than women . . . These sex-specific differences are associated with the finding that postseparation womens' scores are substantially lower than preseparation womens' scores, while the reverse is true in the case of men.'' Bloom and Caldwell (1981) make a very important point when they state: ''Assertions regarding womens' and mens' adjustment to the process of divorce must clearly take into account and control for the point in that process at which the assessment has been made. Studies of couples before or close to the time of separation could well conclude that women have a far more difficult time than men. Studies of persons conducted as shortly as two months after separation could easily come to the opposite conclusion.''

In their study of remarriage after divorce, Spanier and Furstenberg (1982) concluded that ''remarriage after divorce is not associated with enhanced well-being.'' Spanier and Furstenberg report a serendipitous finding of major importance. They state: ''the likelihood of remarriage following divorce may be related to one's well-being during the postseparation period; individuals with the greatest well-being were most likely to be remarried three to five years after their final separation.''

In a study by Berman and Turk (1981), post divorce adjustment was related to the problems encountered after the divorce and the coping strategies utilized in dealing with these problems. The six coping strategies were: Social Activities, Learning, Personal Understanding, Expressing Feelings, Autonomy, and Home and Family Activities. The six problem areas were Former Spouse Contacts, Parent-Child Interactions, Interpersonal Relations, Loneliness, Practical Problems, and Financial Concerns. Berman and Turk maintain that neither coping strategies alone nor the problems encountered by divorced persons could explain or account for adjustment to divorce. Both coping strategies and problem areas are interactive, i.e., neither should be studied in isolation. One interesting result of the regression analysis was that the belief that expressing feelings is helpful to adjustment was correlated with a low level of life satisfaction.

Constance Ahrons has created a conceptual model which views divorce as a crisis of family transition (Ahrons, 1980, 1983). Using family stress theory in league with systems theory, Ahrons has identified five transitions in the divorce process: Individual cognition; Family metacognition; systemic separation; systemic reorganization; and Family redefinition. These transitions usually overlap. Ahrons focuses on the relationships between the former partners: She conceptualizes divorce as a process of family change. When this process fails or is otherwise aborted by an unwilling ex-mate, the degree of recovery and return to a new level of functioning is impaired. The importance of Ahrons work is reflected in the proposition that grief resolution is enhanced when/if the ex-mates can cooperate in their future role (redefined) as coparents. Without such successful transitioning the grief work may be prolonged and labored.

Kenneth Kressel has dealt specifically with the patterns of coping as these patterns carry implications for clinicians (Kressel, 1980). Kressel confirms the lag in recovery of the passive agents compared to the active agents (Kressel uses the terms initiator and noninitiator). Kressel notes that the noninitiator may not recover fully for as long as three years or more after separation. Kressel's four stages are: Denial, Mourning, Anger, Readjustment. Kressel sees these stages as part of a "general human adaptive mechanism." Kressel further sees the coping process as consisting of four major periods: Pre-divorce decision period; Decision period; A period of negotiations; a period of re-equilibration. The study by Kressel drew upon a series of in-depth interviews with over 50 lawyers, judges, psychotherapists, and clergy, together with a study of 17 couples who were participants in a program designed to assist the divorcing spouses in negotiating their divorce settlements.

Sprenkle and Cyrus have summarized the abandonment literature, especially as it is related to therapeutic intervention (Sprenkle and Cyrus, 1983). Likewise, Fulmer (1983) has dealt with the issue of unresolved mourning in single parent families.

OVERVIEW OF PHASE I—PILOT STUDY

Phase One utilized a three stage model of grief resolution: Stage One was the Approach/Avoidance stage, extending from the first serious thoughts about divorce to separation and/or filing. Stage Two was the Separation/Filing stage extending from separation and/or filing to the final divorce decree. Stage Three was the Resolution/Closure stage extending from the final decree to penultimate closure. Within these three stages comparisons were made between the active agents and the passive agents on three types of clusters: Affective or emotional, Cognitive or thought, and Behavioral or activity-related items. The predominant research conclusion was that the active agents in divorce pass through the three stages at a more rapid rate than the passive agents, but that both sets of agents experience a wide range of recurring feelings, thoughts, and behaviors. These recurring patterns are circular even as they proceed in an observable linear direction. The results of the Phase I, (Pilot Study) indicated: (1) The active agent in divorce will more likely be able to bring closure to his/her anger sooner than the passive agent, (2) The active agent will likely begin reconstruction sooner than the passive agent—due to the fact that the active agent had a head start as the result of earlier cognitive acceptance, (3) Negotiation was a predominating behavioral cluster for the passive agent, especially in the second stage, i.e. (from separation or filing to the final decree), this reflects the lag between the active and passive agents, (4) The passive agent in stage three (Resolution-closure: from final decree to penultimate acceptance) continued to deal with the divorce whereas the active agent had done this in stage two, (5) Feelings of failure are more frequent for passive agents in the third stage than they are for active agents.

In all measures, the active agents appeared to negotiate the three stages in a more rapid manner than did the passive agents. We induce the premise that the actives are the initiators of the divorce action (whether or not they are the actual "divorcers" or "filers" is beside the point: a "provoker" is always the active agent even if the provoker's mate is the one who finally files for divorce). Because the active agents are the real initiators it is reasonable to assume that they are ahead of the passive agents in the process of acceptance and resolution.

The data from the first phase of the research indicated that there is most certainly a similarity between the Kubler-Ross model of grief resolution at bereavement due to death and the sequence of feelings, thoughts, and behaviors related to grief resolution following divorce. There is a general progression through the recurring feelings, thoughts, and behavior's which we believe is indeed similar to the grief resolution sequence identified by Kubler-Ross. Nevertheless, pressing the similarity beyond this generic resemblance is an over-simplification due mainly to the very different sets of dynamics and related responsibilities.

The dynamic which differentiates the two grief resolution processes is the decision factor which is almost always present in divorce but is much less present in death. "Except for those situations noted in connection with life-death decisioning, death bereavement lacks the element of decisioning which is the sine qua non to divorce'' (Crosby, Gage, Raymond, 1983). In short, responsibility for one's actions plays a much greater role in the resolution of grief resulting from divorce than it does in the resolution of grief resulting from death. This is not to deny that a sense of guilt and/or failure is a very real factor in bereavement following death. Nevertheless, it is of a different genre when compared to the sense of guilt and/or failure ensuing from divorce. ''Divorce is a decision of major proportion and implication for the more active agent who decides and for the more passive agent who has been left with the inescapable consequences of the active agents' decision'' (Crosby, Gage, Raymond, 1983).

THE SELF-REPORT QUESTIONNAIRE

The instrument utilized in this study was the result of the authors' attempt to ''tease'' out the nature and sequencing of feelings, thoughts, and behaviors associated with the entire divorce process, beginning with the first serious thoughts about divorce and extending to penultimate closure. Whereas the Phase One pilot study invited the respondents to tell their own story in essay form following twelve guideline questions, Phase Two substituted three sets of direct questions. This was done primarily because the Phase One essay accounts proved to be too difficult to reduce to quantitative measurement. Secondly, the essay format of ''telling your own story'' proved, for research purposes, to be self-defeating in that numerous participants withdrew because they found the experience to be too painful.

The creation of an instrument which would capture the identification and sequencing of feelings, thoughts, and behaviors was a challenging task, howbeit questionable in terms of internal validity (i.e., Does the experience of responding to the items serve to sensitize the respondent? To what degree is recall impaired by later success in rebuilding one's life? Is the universe of feelings, thoughts, and behaviors adequately summarized in the questionnaire?).

The first part of the questionnaire consisted of sixteen questions relating to demographics and biography. These questions serve to determine the respondent's age, number of divorces, length of marriages, number of children, marital union to which the children were born, birth order of respondent, years since divorce was final, S.E.S. data, religious preference, gender identification, and educational level.

The second part of the questionnaire consisted of twenty-nine questions. These questions relate to the realization, consideration, and discussion of divorce; the initiation of discussion; the emerging likelihood of divorce; avoidance, blocking out, denial; attempts at compromise, accommodation, and reconciliation; the handling and expression of anger, guilt, and a sense of failure; recognition and dealing with depression; the presence or absence of counseling and type of counseling; results of counseling; other emotional support systems; feelings of aloneness; separation-reuniting-separation patterns; feelings, thoughts, and behavior's related to a sense of release, relief, and/or extrication from a destructive situation together with feelings related to reduced stress and conflict; and points of progress toward resolution and acceptance.

The third part of the instrument was a single question structured as a taxonomy wherein the respondent was asked to classify the strength and/or prevalence of a thought, feeling, or behavior. The question listed twenty events including awareness of the problem, denial, efforts to negotiate, accommodation, announcements of intention to carry through with the divorce, separation, post-separation, finality of decree, rebuilding new lifestyle, coping, and adjustment to singlehood and the possibility of future remarriage. Each of the twenty events was to be responded to in three ways—with a feeling response, a thought response, and a behavioral response. The selection of responses is limited. There are fourteen possible affective responses to choose from for each of the twenty events. There are eleven possible cognitive responses to choose from for each of the twenty events. There are thirteen possible behavioral responses to choose from for each of the twenty events. In short, the taxonomy calls for a total of sixty responses to be chosen from a list of affective, cognitive, and behavioral possibilities.

The precise tracking and ordering of these responses is intended to reveal the path toward resolution and acceptance of the individual respondent. Taken collectively, the patterns and trends of the finding's indicate the nature of the resolution process.

The questionnaire also afforded the respondent an opportunity to make final personal comments related to the respondent's feeling as he/she completed the questionnaire. The researchers hoped that this would allow for the expression of widely divergent material and perhaps lead to serendipitous insights regarding the process of grief resolution.

SUBJECT CHARACTERISTICS

Approximately three hundred persons volunteered to participate in the study. Two hundred questionnaires were received. Of these 59 were unusable. This study is based on 141 persons. Females numbered 108 and males 33. Male representation constituted slightly less than 25 percent (23.4). In terms of actives, passives, and mutuals in the making of the decision to divorce, the actives numbered 56, the passives 42, and the mutuals 43. The modal age of the male participants was 31–35 years of age (12) with 23 of the 33 males being between 31 and 45 years of age. The modal age of the female participants was identical to the males, 31–35 (32) with 92 of the 108 females being between 26 and 45 years of age. Fourteen of the 33 males were 41 years old or older. Thirty of the 108 females were 41 years old or older. This is a contrasting percentage of 42.4% males over 40 to 27.8% females over 40.

Total sample birth order of the divorcing persons indicated that first borns were more likely to be active agents (N = 21) versus 11 passive agents and 16 mutual agents. Last born children were more likely to be either passive agents (N = 15) or mutual agents (N = 12). Middle borns demonstrated a greater frequency of active agents (N = 17) than passive agents (N = 4) or mutuals (N = 12). Among the males the last borns displayed twice the frequency of being passive agents compared to being active agents or mutual agents (N = 6, N = 3, N = 3). Among the females the first borns displayed twice the frequency of being active agents compared to being passive agents and one third greater frequency than mutual agents. (Active first born females, N = 18; passive first-born females, N = 8; mutual first born females N = 12). Middle born females also displayed twice the frequency in being active agents versus passive and mutual (N = 17, N = 9, N = 7).

Among the 141 participants, 139 were reporting the experience of divorce following first marriage, only two persons reported the divorce experience following a second marriage. The duration of all marriages ranged from less than one year to over 26 years. The modal point was 6–10 years duration. (One third: 47 out of 141.) This mode held for actives, passives, and mutuals. Of the total sample, 45 participants (31.9%) had no children, 30 participants (21.3%) had one child, and 43 participants (30.5%) had two children. Twenty-three participants (16.3%) had more than two children. All children belonged to the 139 first divorce participants. An almost equal number of actives (N = 15), passives (N = 16), and mutuals (N = 15) had no children. The number of active participants with one child was twice the number of combined passives and mutuals. Actives and passives with two children were both nearly twice as many as the mutuals (N = 17, 17, 9).

When both husband and wife were employed full time there was a total of 49 divorces (34.8%) (actives N = 20, passives N = 14, mutuals N = 15). When only the husband was gainfully employed there were 21 divorces fairly evenly distributed (7, 8, 6). With husband full time and wife part time there were 28 divorces (10, 9, 9), and when the wife returned to work after being at home there were 12 divorces (6, 2, 4). Among a category labelled "other" we found a combination of husbands who were students, with wives who worked. This group accounted for 31 divorces (13, 9, 9), the second largest group.

The sample proved to be overwhelmingly waspish. Ninety-eight divorces were amongst protestants (actives 37, passives 30, mutuals 31). Twenty-nine were among Roman Catholics (9, 10, 10). There were no Jewish participants, 6 Unitarians, 4 non or no religion, and 4 "other." All participants were caucasian.

FAILURE-GUILT-DEPRESSION-MEANING

A noteworthy result points to the reality of a sense of failure, guilt, depression among actives, passives, and mutuals. Related to this is the return of a sense of meaning in one's life.

The sense of failure was strong across all three groups, i.e., actives, passives, and mutuals. Twenty-one actives expressed strong feelings of having failed. (Actives: no failure N = 10, slight failure N = 9, medium failure N = 16, strong failure N = 21). Among the passives over half expressed strong failure (none N = 4, slight N = 6, medium N = 10, strong N = 22). Among the mutuals the pattern was similar (none N = 6, slight N = 6, medium N = 13, strong N = 18). Combining the medium and strong reactions across actives, passives, and mutuals reveals that 100 subjects felt medium to strong feelings of failure (medium 27.7%; strong 43.3%).

A strong sense of guilt was expressed by 36.9% of all respondents. Twenty-five actives expressed strong feelings of guilt (none N = 12, slight N = 11, medium N = 8, strong N = 25). Among passives, however, 15 expressed no feelings of guilt (even though 22 had expressed strong feelings of failure). Twelve passives expressed strong guilt feelings (none N = 15, slight N = 5, medium N = 10, strong N = 12). Mutuals maintained the modal point of the actives (none N = 9, slight N = 11, medium N = 8, and strong N = 15). Taken across the three groups, 52 (36.9%) persons expressed strong guilt and 36 (25.5%) expressed no guilt, leaving 53 (37.6%) in the middle range.

Thirteen persons reported no depression throughout the entire experience (actives N = 7, passives N = 1, mutuals N = 5). For the remaining 128 subjects depression was modal at the beginning of the divorce process and in the middle of the process with a distinct lessening as the process moved toward the decree stage. This held for all three groups. For all three groups there were 42 subjects reporting the strongest depression at the beginning of the process (actives N = 16, passives N = 10, mutuals N = 16). Thirty-five subjects felt the strongest depression midway in the process (actives N = 16, passive N = 11, mutuals N = 8). The other 51 subjects experienced the strongest depression at the time near the final decree and following the final decree.

In answer to the question: "How much time elapsed from the final decree until your life became more meaningful?" the actives and mutuals revealed a modal point of "immediately." The passives, however, showed a mode of from one to two years. Seven reported that they had not yet experienced a return of meaning (actives N = 1, passives N = 5, mutuals N = 1). Across the three groups there were 38 persons (27%) who reported the return of meaning immediately after the divorce was final (actives N = 19, passives N = 6, mutuals N = 13). The next highest mode across groups was the one-to-two years interval (actives N = 14, passives N = 12, mutuals N = 7). The third highest mode was the 6 months-to-one year interval (actives N = 12, passives N = 5, mutuals N = 7). A total of 16 persons reported that it took more than 5 years before their life became more meaningful (actives N = 4, passives N = 4, mutuals N = 8).

That portion of the subjects (N = 93, 66.4%) which entered counseling or therapy reported an increase in positive feelings toward self as the primary benefit of the experience. Actives, passives, and mutuals predominately sought counseling for themselves, rather than for the mate or for the dyad. The actives sought counseling primarily after they first gave serious consideration to divorce. The passives sought counseling primarily after the divorce was final. The mutuals sought counseling primarily prior to consideration of divorce. Of the 93 persons who sought counseling, there were 34 actives, 33 passives, and 26 mutuals.

RESULTS

Figure 1 represents the various clusters of affect, cognition, and behavior. Each cluster carries a name under which is subsumed an entire range of related feelings, thoughts, or behaviors. For example the affective cluster of anger includes anger, hostility, resentment, hate, rage, bitterness, pique, irritation, and annoyance. The name or banner word for each cluster is the word employed in the analysis of the data: This banner word is always to be understood as representative of the various words listed under the banner word in Figure 1.

STAGE ONE: FIRST AWARENESS OF SERIOUS MARITAL PROBLEMS

In the first stage of the process 9 of the active agents (N = 56) listed their primary affective response as fear (33.9%). The second most frequent response was hurt (N = 18; 32.1%). These two responses, when combined, constitute 66% of the total active subjects on the variable of affect. The active agents listed approach as the predominant first response in the cognitive clusters (N = 25; 44.6%). The second most frequent response was avoidance (N = 15; 26.8%). In the behavioral cluster the active agents again listed approach as the modal response (N = 29; 51.8%). The next most frequent responses were avoidance (N = 10) and reconstruction (N = 8). The stage one data analysis on actives, or affect, cognition and behavior revealed a Chi Square significant at .001 on each variable.

In the first stage of the process 18 of the passive agents (N = 42) listed their primary affective response as hurt (32.9%). The next most frequent affective responses were apathy (N = 9) and fear (N = 7). The passive agents listed avoidance as the modal response in the cognitive clusters (N = 21; 50%). The next most frequent responses were approach (N = 10) and ambivalence (N = 8). In

Affective Clusters	Cognitive Clusters	Behavioral Clusters
Anger	**Approach**	**Approach**
Anger	Approach	Approach
Hostility	Reconsideration	Reconsider
Resentment	Consideration	Consider
Hate	Entertaining ideas	Moving toward
Rage	and alternatives	Level
Bitterness	Thinking about differ-	Confront
Pique	ences, trust, attrac-	Initiate
Irritation	tions, wants, needs	Sex: hi-demand
Annoyance	assurance	Express anger
		Express hurt
Hurt	**Avoidance**	Separate
Hurt	Avoidance	File
Pain	Denial	
Sadness	Repress	**Avoidance**
Grief	Suppress	Avoidance
Mourning	Block-out	Procrastinate
Disappointment	Sublimation	Run away
Rejection	Escape	Escape
Lost	Take rather than give	Repress
Abandoned	If I don't face it, it	Suppress
	will go away	Block-out
Despair	It isn't true	Moving-away
Despair	It can't happen	Detach
Hopeless	It won't happen	Ignore requests of
Shattered		mate
Devastated	**Ambivalence**	Physical symptoms
Desolate	Ambivalence	Interrupt mate
Futility	Approach-Avoidance	Contradict mate
Depressed	Avoidance-Approach	Label
Overwhelmed	Indecisive	Argumentative
Alone	Procrastinate	Affairs
Loneliness	Wishy-Washy	Sex-no interest
Self-pity	On the fence	Eyes cast down
Desperate	Immobilized	Succinct speech
Bewildered	Double-bind	Passive-Aggressive
Shock	Caught	
	Trapped	**Negotiate**
Apathy		Negotiate
Apathy	**Acceptance**	Compromise
Numb	Acceptance	Congruent-level
Indifferent	Realize self-power	Bargain
Ennui	Understanding	Accommodate
Malaise	Comprehension	Compliance
	Empathy with mate	Conciliatory
	Equitable division of	Placate
	responsibility & blame	Quid Pro Quo
		Trade-offs
Fear	**Analysis**	**Acceptance**
Fear	Analyze feelings	Acceptance
Afraid	Analyze failure	Toleration
Apprehensive	Analyze guilt	Distancing
Worry	Re-analyze	Separation
Anxiety	Doubt earlier conclu-	Integration
Scared	sions and decisions	Re-defining
Dread	Introspection	Resolve
Tense	Integration	
Uncertainty	Redefinition	

FIGURE 1. Clusters of Affect, Cognition, and Behavior

Affective Clusters	Cognitive Clusters	Behavioral Clusters
Failure	Reorientation	Reconstruct
Failure	Individualism	Reconstruct
Guilt	Mental closure	Rebuild
Inadequate	(penultimate)	Dating
Incompetent		Working
Self-recrimination		Learning
Low self-esteem		Trust self
Low self-worth		Love self
Inferiority		Respect self
Frustration		Approve self
		Affirm self
Hope		Assert self
Hope		Accept self
Free		Believe in self
Relief		Re-orientation
Release		Re-defining
Glad		Testing out behavior
Happy		Individuation
Joyful		Integration
Optimistic		Regain equilibrium
High self-esteem		Behavioral closure
High self-worth		(penultimate)
We can make it		
We can work it out		

FIGURE 1, continued

the behavioral cluster the passive agents listed approach as the modal response (N = 18; 32.9%). The next most frequent responses were negotiation (N = 10), acceptance (N = 8), and avoidance (N = 6). The stage one data analysis of passives on affect, cognition, and behavior revealed a chi square significant at .001 on each variable.

In the first stage of the process 15 of the mutual agents (N = 43) listed their primary affective response as fear (34.9%), followed closely by hurt (N = 12; 27.9%). The mutual agents listed approach as the modal response in the cognitive clusters (N = 17; 39.5%). Acceptance, ambivalence, and avoidance followed with 8, 7, and 7 respectively. In the behavioral cluster the mutual agents again listed approach as the modal response (N = 23; 53.5%). All other responses were fairly evenly distributed (negotiation N = 6, avoidance N = 5, reconstruction N = 5, and acceptance N = 4). The stage one data analysis of mutuals revealed a chi square significant at .001 on the affect and behavior variables and .05 on the cognition variable.

STAGE TWO: SEPARATION OR FILING

In the second stage of the process 22 of the active agents (N = 56) listed their primary affective response as hope (39.3%). The second most frequent affective response was fear (N = 12; 21.4%). The active agents listed acceptance as the modal response in the cognitive clusters (N = 31; 55.4%), followed by approach (N = 11) and analysis (N = 8). In the behavioral cluster the active agents listed reconstruction as the modal response (N = 27; 48.2%), followed by acceptance (N = 10) and avoidance (N = 9). The stage two data analysis of actives on affect, cognition, and behavior revealed a significant chi square at .001 on each variable.

In the second stage of the process 11 of the passive agents (N = 42) listed their primary affective response as hurt (26.2%) with fear as the next most frequent response (N = 10; 23.8%). The passive agents listed acceptance (N = 10), ambivalence (N = 9), approach (N = 9), and avoidance (N = 9) as responses in the cognitive clusters. In the behavioral cluster the passive agents listed negotiation as the modal response (N = 15; 35.7%) followed by acceptance (N = 12; 28.6%). The stage two data analysis of passives revealed a chi square significant at .05 on the variables of affect and behavior. Data on cognition was not statistically significant.

In the second stage of the process the mutual agents (N = 43) listed their primary affective response in a tri-modal pattern. Hope (N = 11) was followed closely by fear (N = 10) and hurt (N = 10). The mutual agents listed acceptance as the modal first response in the cognitive clusters (N = 22; 51.2%). The second most frequent response was analysis (N = 9; 20.9%). In the behavioral cluster the mutual agents were bi-modal in their responses. Reconstruction and acceptance were the response of 13 persons (combined N = 26; 60.05%). The stage two data analysis of mutuals revealed a chi square significant at .05 on the affect variable and a chi square significant at .001 on the cognition variable. Data on behavior was not statistically significant.

STAGE THREE: FINAL DECREE

In the third stage of the process 38 of the active agents (N = 56) listed their primary affective response as hope (67.9%) with no decisive modes among the other responses. The active agents listed acceptance as the modal response in the cognitive clusters (N=30; 53.6%). The second most frequent response was analysis (N = 21; 37.5%). In the behavioral cluster the active agents listed reconstruction as the modal response (N = 43; 76.8%) with acceptance being the second most frequent response (N = 8; 14.3%) The stage three data analysis of actives on affect, cognition, and behavior revealed a chi square significant at .001 on each variable.

In the third stage of the process 15 of the passive agents (N = 42) listed their primary affective response as hope (35.7%) with hurt (N = 8) and despair (N = 5) and fear (N = 5) following. The passive agents listed acceptance as the modal response in the cognitive clusters (N = 20; 47.6%). The secondary mode was analysis (N = 9; 21.4%). In the behavioral cluster the passive agents listed reconstruction as the modal response (N = 25; 59.5%). This was followed by acceptance (N = 9; 21.4%). The stage three data analysis of passives revealed a chi square significant at .05 on the affect variable and a chi square significant at .001 on the cognition and behavior variables.

In the third stage of the process 24 of the mutual agents (N = 43) listed their primary affective response as hope (55.8%). The mutual agents listed acceptance as the modal response in the cognitive clusters (N = 27; 62.8%). The secondary mode was analysis (N = 9). In the behavioral cluster the mutual agents listed reconstruction as the modal response (N = 30; 69.8%). The next most frequent response was acceptance (N = 6). The stage three data analysis of mutuals on affect, cognition, and behavior revealed a chi square significant at .001 on each variable.

Figure 2 represents the frequency of response for each variable by actives, passives, and mutuals over the three successives stages.

DISCUSSION

When the number and percentage of responses indicating modal trends is combined with the use of chi square, there emerges a pattern of grief resolution in divorce. This pattern remains unclear at two points, i.e., the stage two passives on cognition and the stage two mutuals on behavior. At five points the probability of obtaining similar results by chance is five out of one hundred (.05). The remaining 20 chi squares revealed a probability of one per thousand (.001).

An overview of the pattern reveals the active agents as experiencing fear, hope, and hope in the three stage affective progression; approach, acceptance, and acceptance in the three stage cognitive progression; and approach, reconstruction, and reconstruction in the three stage behavioral progression.

	Active Agents N=56			Passive Agents N=42			Mutual Agents N=43		
	Affective	Cognitive	Behavioral	Affective	Cognitive	Behavioral	Affective	Cognitive	Behavioral
Stage 1. First Awareness of Serious Marital Problems	Fear 19	Approach 25	Approach 29	Hurt 18	Avoidance 21	Approach 18	Fear 15	Approach 17	Approach 23
	Hurt 18	Avoidance 15	Avoidance 10	Apathy 9	Approach 10	Negotiation 10	Hurt 12	Acceptance 8	Negotiation 6
	Anger 7	Ambivalence 9	Reconstru- tion 8	Fear 7	Ambivalence 8	Acceptance 8	Anger 5	Ambivalence 7	Avoidance 5
	Failure 7	Acceptance 4	Negotiation 6	Failure 4	Acceptance 2	Avoidance 6	Failure 5	Avoidance 7	Reconstruc- tion 5
	Despair 3	Analysis 3	Acceptance 3	Hope 2	Analysis 1	Reconstruc- tion 0	Apathy 3	Analysis 4	Acceptance 4
	Apathy 1			Anger 1			Despair 3		
	Hope 1			Despair 1			Hope 0		
	$X^2=43.25$ p=.001 6df	$X^2=29.3$ p=.001 4df	$X^2=37.73$ p=.001 4df	$X^2=37.35$ p=.001 6df	$X^2=30.62$ p=.001 4df	$X^2=20.38$ p=.001 4df	$X^2=27.88$ p=.001 6df	$X^2=11.29$ p=.05 4df	$X^2=30.39$ p=.001 4df
Stage 2. Separation or Filing	Hope 22	Acceptance 31	Reconstruc- tion 27	Hurt 11	Acceptance 10	Negotiation 15	Hope 11	Acceptance 22	Reconstruc- tion 13
	Fear 12	Approach 11	Acceptance 10	Fear 10	Ambivalence 9	Acceptance 12	Fear 10	Analysis 9	Acceptance 13
	Apathy 6	Analysis 8	Avoidance 9	Apathy 6	Approach 9	Reconstruc- tion 7	Hurt 10	Approach 6	Avoidance 7
	Hurt 6	Avoidance 5	Approach 7	Despair 6	Avoidance 9	Approach 5	Despair 4	Avoidance 4	Approach 7
	Anger 4	Ambivalence 1	Negotiation 3	Anger 5	Analysis 5	Avoidance 3	Failure 4	Ambivalence 2	Negotiation 3
	Failure 4			Hope 3			Apathy 3		
	Despair 2			Failure 1			Anger 1		
	$X^2=36$ p=.001 6df	$X^2=48.63$ p=.001 4df	$X^2=30.43$ p=.001 4df	$X^2=12.68$ p=.05 6df	$X^2=1.8$ N.S. 4df	$X^2=11.8$ p=.05 4df	$X^2=15.95$ p=.05 6df	$X^2=29.2$ p=.001 4df	$X^2=7.17$ N.S. 4df
Stage 3. Final Decree	Hope 38	Acceptance 30	Reconstruc- tion 43	Hope 15	Acceptance 20	Reconstruc- tion 25	Hope 24	Acceptance 27	Reconstruc- tion 30
	Apathy 6	Analysis 21	Acceptance 8	Hurt 8	Analysis 9	Acceptance 9	Hurt 6	Analysis 9	Acceptance 6
	Fear 5	Approach 2	Avoidance 3	Despair 5	Avoidance 6	Negotiation 4	Fear 5	Approach 3	Avoidance 3
	Failure 4	Avoidance 2	Approach 1	Fear 5	Approach 5	Avoidance 4	Apathy 4	Avoidance 3	Negotiation 3
	Hurt 2	Ambivalence 1	Negotiation 1	Anger 3	Ambivalence 2	Approach 0	Anger 3	Ambivalence 1	Approach 1
	Anger 1			Apathy 3			Failure 1		
	Despair 0			Failure 3			Despair 0		
	$X^2=134.75$ p=.001 6df	$X^2=64.55$ p=.001 4df	$X^2=115.78$ p=.001 4df	$X^2=19.01$ p=.05 6df	$X^2=23$ p=.001 4df	$X^2=31.94$ p=.001 4df	$X^2=64.33$ p=.001 6df	$X^2=53.41$ p=.001 4df	$X^2=68.06$ p=.001 4df

X^2 .05 6df = 12.59; X^2 .05 4df = 9.49; X^2 .001 6df = 22.46; X^2 .001 4df = 18.46

FIGURE 2. Frequency of Response per Cluster by Agents and by Stage

The pattern with the passive agents reveals hurt, hurt, and hope in the three stage affective progression; avoidance, (mixed pattern),* and acceptance in the three stage cognitive progression; and approach, negotiation, and reconstruction in the three stage behavioral progression.

The pattern with the mutual agents reveals fear, hope, and hope in the three stage affective progression; approach, acceptance, and acceptance in the three stage cognitive progression; and approach (reconstruction/acceptance),* and reconstruction in the three stage behavior progression.

The flow of the pattern appears to be consistent within the differing experiences of the actives, passives, and mutuals. We would expect active agents to recover more quickly than passives (Crosby, 1983) if for no other reason than they have an edge in feeling, thinking, and acting (behaving) about the divorce decision. While the active agents are feeling fear in stage two, the passives are still predominantly feeling hurt. It is interesting that both the actives and passives are feeling hope in stage three, although the mode and chi square for the actives is more predominant than for the passives.

The actives and passives think differently in stage one. The actives are thinking primarily approach while the passives are thinking avoidance. In stage two the actives are thinking acceptance and the passives give no clear picture. In stage three both the actives and passives are thinking acceptance.

The actives and passives behave alike in stage one. They both seek to approach. In stage two, however, the actives are busy at reconstruction while the passives are attempting to negotiate. By stage three both the actives and the passives are attempting reconstruction.

The 1983 pilot study did not include the consideration of mutuals. Except for the stage two mutuals' behavior (bi-modal; reconstruction and acceptance) the mutuals are identical in all other ways to the actives. This finding would appear to be consistent with a so-called common-sense analysis, in that mutuals, however, distraught, hurt, angry, or despairing, have come to a mutual decision. This mutuality also does not imply a strictly fifty-fifty balance but it does imply that the decision had been made by two participants rather than unilaterally. We would expect the mutuals to differ from the passives, who had the decision made for them by the actives.

The 1983 pilot study based on first hand autobiographical

---

*Parents indicate a non-significant chi-square at .05.

accounts of seventeen divorced persons indicated a definite lag of the passives in stage two and extending into stage three. The present study does not reveal the lagging into stage three as was indicated in the pilot study. Certainly the differential between actives and passives is clear at stage two. In this sense, one of the most important conclusions of the 1983 study was the existence of a lag continuing into the third stage (final decree and after). This lag is not confirmed or upheld in our present sample. One explanation for this major difference is that by the time the final stage became reality, the passives had somehow caught up! They had more ground to cover in stage two and they succeeded in the task. Another possible explanation is, of course, that the research instrument was not sensitive enough to tap into a possible passive lag as they entered stage three.

CONCLUSIONS

After completing the pilot study and with the publication herein of findings using a much larger sample, what may be said with confidence about the grief resolution process in divorce?

First, a comparison with eight other models (Crosby, 1983) and with several models mentioned in the literature review of this study, suggests that while other paradigms, conceptual frameworks, or models have attractive components and justifications, the three stage model with three distinct sets of filing categories on the three variables of affect, cognition, and behavior is a clear and parsimonious model. The $3 \times 3 \times 3$ framework allows for the expression of change, progression, and regression. It allows for circular as well as linear interpretations. Finally, it permits a frame by which comparisons and contrasts may be drawn. The use of clusters (Figure 1) in this study proved to be convenient and expedient in that semantical economy, perceptual clarity, and parsimony are more easily attainable.

The greatest question, still unresolved in our mind, is the need for an instrument which allows for meaningful self report and fulfills the requirements for reliability, validity, and general comprehensiveness. It should be noted that the 1983 pilot utilized personal essay-type accounts of one's journey through the grief resolution process. This type of instrument proved to be extremely difficult for both the person telling his/her own story and for the reader-researcher attempting to analyze the account. The instrument utilized in the present study proved to be cumbersome. We have yet to establish any coefficients of reliability or concurrent validity.

Male representation proved to be a disappointment (N = 33; 23.4%) of total respondents (N = 141). In this light, our results can be interpreted as applying to females more than to males. We still await a more viable instrument and a more balanced sex ratio in a larger sample.

The 1983 pilot served to establish the clusters (Figure 1). This second stage effort serves to differentiate which clusters predominate using the three stages, three agents, and three variables. The challenge now becomes one of utilizing the conceptual model (3 × 3 × 3) and the clusters in such a manner as to test future samples against the patterns revealed in our present data. For this purpose we seek improved instrumentation and a larger, random sample. Concurrent and construct validity could be tested by utilizing the 3 × 3 × 3 model with the clusters of figure one in various other instrument modes, such as personal interviews, semi-projective use of vignettes, and self-report rank ordering procedures.

Aside from the use of the 3 × 3 × 3 model and the use of clusters to afford semantic and perceptual clarity, the overriding research implication is that grief resolution in the process of divorce is circular, recurring in intensity, and dependent on many factors such as active, passive, or mutual agent; duration of marriage, age, presence and age of children. Clinical implications include the truism that "normal" is a very broad and diverse range of feelings, thoughts, and behaviors. Abnormal grief reaction is perhaps more readily and easily conceptualized and operationalized. Perhaps the most significant contribution of all divorce—grief research is the increasing confidence with which we may label, define, or reframe grief as being "normal," healthy, and necessary for recovery, acceptance, and the business of reconstructing one's future.

REFERENCES

Ahrons, C. R. (1980). Divorce: A crisis of family transition and change. *Family Relations, 29* (4) 533–540.

Ahrons, C. R. (1983). Divorce: Before, during and after. In H. McCubbin & C. R. Figley (Eds.), *Stress and the Family*. N. Y.: Brunner/Mazel.

Albrecht, S. L., Kunz, P. R. (1980). The decision to divorce: a social exchange perspective. *Journal of Divorce, 3* (4) 319–337.

Berman, W. H., Turk, D. C. (1981). Adaptation to divorce: problems and coping strategies. *Journal of Marriage and the Family, 43* (1) 179–189.

Bloom, B. L., Caldwell, R. A. (1981). Sex differences in adjustment during the process of marital separation. *Journal of Marriage and the Family, 43* (3) 693–701.

Bohannan, P. (1970). The six stations of divorce. In P. Bohannan (Ed.), *Divorce and After*. Garden City, N. Y.: Doubleday.

Brown, P., Felton, B. J., Whiteman, V., & Manela, R. (1980). Attachment and distress following marital separation. *Journal of Divorce, 3* (4) 303–317.

Crosby, J., Gage, B., Raymond, M. (1983). The Grief Resolution Process in Divorce, *Journal of Divorce, 7* (1) 3–18.

Daniels-Mohring, D., Berger, M. (1984). Social network changes and the adjustment to divorce. *Journal of Divorce, 8* (1) 17–32.

Dasteel, J. D. (1982). Stress reactions to marital dissolution as experienced by adults attending courses on divorce. *Journal of Divorce, 5* (3) 37–47.

Davenport, D. S. (1981). A closer look at the 'healthy' grieving process. *The Personnel and Guidance Journal, 59* (6) 332f.

Davidoff, I. F., Schiller, M. S. (1983). The divorce workshop as a crisis intervention: A practical model. *Journal of Divorce, 6* (4) 37–54.

Defazio, V. J., Kleinbort, I. (1975). A note on the dynamics of psychotherapy during marital dissolution. *Psychotherapy: Theory and Practice, 12*, 101–104.

Frears, L. H., Schneider, J. M. (1981). Exploring loss and grief within a wholistic framework. *The Personnel and Guidance Journal, 59* (6) 341f.

Fulmer, R. H. (1983). A structural approach to unresolved mourning in single parent family systems. *Journal of Marriage and Family Therapy, 9* (3) 259–269.

Hancock E. (1980). The dimensions of meaning and belonging in the process of divorce. *American Journal of Orthopsychiatry, 50* (1) 18–27.

Heikkinen C. A. (1981). Loss resolution for growth. *The Personnel and Guidance Journal, 59* (6) 327f.

Herman, S. J. (1974). Divorce: a grief process. *Perspectives in Psychiatric Care. 12*, 108–112.

Kaslow, F. W. (1984). Divorce: an evolutionary process of change in the family system. *Journal of Divorce, 7* (3) 21–39.

Kessler, S. (1975). *The American Way of Divorce*. Chicago: Nelson-Hall.

Kitson, G. C., Sussman, M. B. (1983). Marital complaints, demographic characteristics, and symptoms of mental distress in divorce. *Journal of Marriage and the Family, 45* (1) 103–113.

Kitson, G. C. (1982). Attachment to the spouse in divorce: a scale and its application. *Journal of Marriage and the Family, 44* (2) 379–393.

Kolevzon, M. S., Gottlieb, S. J. (1983). The impact of divorce: a multivariate study. *Journal of Divorce, 7* (2), 89–98.

Kraus, S. (1979): The crisis of divorce: growth promoting or pathogenic? *Journal of Divorce, 3* (2) 107–119.

Kressel, K. Deutsch, M. (1977). Divorce therapy: an in-depth survey of therapists' views. *Family Process, 16* (4) 413–443.

Kressel, K. (1980). Patterns of coping in divorce and some implications for clinical practice. *Family Relations, 29* (2) 234–240.

Saul, S. C., Scherman, A. (1984). Divorce grief and personal adjustment in divorced persons who remarry or remain single. *Journal of Divorce, 7* (3) 75–85.

Spanier, G., Furstenberg, F. (1982). Remarriage after divorce: a longitudinal analysis of well being. *Journal of Marriage and the Family, 44* (3) 709–720.

Spanier, G. B., Thompson, L. (1983). Relief and distress after marital separation. *Journal of Divorce, 7* (1) 31–49.

Spivey, P. B., Scherman, A. (1980). The effects of time lapse on personality characteristics and stress on divorced women. *Journal of Divorce, 4* (1) 49–59.

Sprenkle, D., Cyrus, C. (1983). Abandonment: the stress of sudden divorce. In H. McCubbin and C. R. Figley (Eds.), *Stress and the Family*. N. Y.: Brunner/Mazel.

Stack, S. (1980). The effects of marital dissolution on suicide. *Journal of Marriage and the Family, 42* (1) 83–92.

Thompson, L., Spanier, G. (1983). The end of marriage and acceptance of marital termination. *Journal of Marriage and the Family, 45* (1) 103–113.

Waller, W. (1951). *The Family: a dynamic interpretation*. (R. Hill, revision). New York: Holt, Rinehart & Winston. (Originally published 1938.)

Wasserman, I. M. (1984). A longitudinal analysis of the linkage between suicide, unemployment, and marital dissolution. *Journal of Marriage and the Family, 46* (4) 853–859.

Wiseman, R. S. (1975). Crisis theory and the process of divorce. *Social Casework, 56* (4) 205–212.

Woodward, J. C., Zabel, J., Decosta, C. (1980). Loneliness and divorce. *Journal of Divorce, 4* (1), 73–82.

Zeiss, A. M. Zeiss, R. A., Johnson, S. M. (1980). Sex differences in initiation of and adjustment to divorce. *Journal of Divorce, 4* (2) 21–33.

Divorce: Three Different Experiences for Three Different Families

Carol Masheter

ABSTRACT. This discussion first briefly addresses the utility of Kantor and Lehr's three family types for the study of divorce. Second, definitions of the key terms used in the discussion follow, including Kantor and Lehr's three family types in their ideal and flawed forms. Third, the discussion traces a "trajectory," or course, for each family type from factors leading to divorce through plausible postdivorce responses, including both strengths and vulnerabilities. Finally, the discussion closes with implications and conclusions from these trajectories for the treatment and study of families who divorce.

Common sense tells us that people experience divorce differently. They divorce for different reasons and adapt after divorce differently. With the exception of studies on demographic differences, however, most research implies that divorced persons go through a single, universal process. Alternatively, researchers tend to consider only certain aspects of divorce in isolation from others, i.e., alleged causes separate from alleged consequences. This discussion departs from these predominant views in three ways. First, it considers divorce in terms of the family rather than the isolated individual. Second, it considers differences among families in terms of Kantor and Lehr's three family typologies. Third, the discussion provides an overview of the complexity and diversity of the divorce experience, as it takes each family type through divorce, starting with each family's typical functioning, followed by disruptions which could lead to divorce, and postdivorce adaptations. Consideration of divorce in terms of Kantor and Lehr's family types

---

Carol Masheter, MA, is a PhD candidate, School of Family Studies, University of Connecticut, Storrs, CT 06268.

compliments sociological research on demographic differences and psychological research on the individual who experiences divorce.

UTILITY OF KANTOR AND LEHR'S FAMILY TYPES IN CONSIDERING DIVORCE

Kantor and Lehr (1975) describe three different family types, their values, and styles of interaction. The family types' values and styles of interaction influence individual family members' perception and behavior. Kantor and Lehr consider the strengths and vulnerabilities of each family type in terms of its characteristic core purpose, values, and dysfunctional patterns. This view contrasts with the implicit or explicit suggestion that one type of family is "the healthiest" or "the ideal" (Constantine, 1983) against which all families should measure themselves—or be measured by professionals, such as therapists or researchers. Though Kantor and Lehr's work does not discuss divorce, the notion of more than one way to be healthy—or dysfunctional—provides a useful perspective from which to consider different families' experience of divorce.

DEFINITIONS

According to Kantor and Lehr (1975), each family type (closed, open, and random) strives toward its core purpose through three ideals (affect, power, and meaning) and three access variables (time, space, and energy). In place of definitions, Kantor and Lehr give elaborate descriptions of each family type in terms of these ideals and access variables plus "sketches," e.g., illustrative cases based on actual families who participated in Kantor and Lehr's research. For this discussion, definitions of the family types consist of summaries of Kantor and Lehr's descriptions.[1]

Briefly, the *closed* family prefers stability to change collective family goals to individual choices, values tradition, authority, and emotional reserve, and tends to regard outside information and non-family persons with caution. In contrast, the *random* family prefers change to stability, individual freedom of expression and action to collective goals, paradox and creativity to tradition and rules. The *open* family attempts to balance stability and change, individual and collective interests, seeks and welcomes information and outsiders, and prides itself with democratic decision-making and open expression of feelings (Kantor & Lehr, 1975; Constantine, 1983).[2]

According to Kantor and Lehr (1975), when any of the three family types fails to achieve its core purpose, the type becomes "flawed." The authors suggest that emergence of a flawed family type is symptomatic of a family experiencing serious crisis.[3] A crisis is a temporary, time-limited disruption which must resolve itself one way or another in terms of better than, return to, or worse than pre-crisis functioning (Caplan, 1964; Erikson, 1959). Divorce, or the legal dissolution of marriage, has been conceptualized predominantly as a "disastrous" personal crisis, often resulting in worse than pre-crisis functioning, and more recently as a "growth-promoting" crisis which can lead to better than pre-crisis functioning (Kraus, 1979).

When overwhelmed by a crisis, such as divorce, most families, regardless of type, intensify their usual, functional strategies. If these usual strategies fail, they can become exaggerated to the point of parody and ironically can become part of the problem (Watzlawick, Weakland & Fisch, 1974). For example, when confronted with crisis, the closed family tends to seal itself off from the outside world, forestalls evolution and change, and attempts to remain the same in spite of the onrush of time. The "benign dictatorship" of tradition and the parents' unquestioned authority become oppressive. Trapped without relief or escape, the family members become lonely and frustrated. However, the closed family's limited range of acceptable affective expression either forces family members to withdraw into depression or to lash out in unacceptable displays of pain and anger (Kantor & Lehr, 1975).

The random family, when confronted with crisis, becomes truly chaotic. Events become incomprehensible and irrelevant; family members risk losing their grasp on meaning. Emotions exceed ecstasy, overflowing into unrestrained fervor. Members are stranded with their feelings without recognition or validation. Frequent and furious fights are the only alternative to alienation. Intense competition can result; physical strength is the frequent and final arbiter of disputes. Kantor and Lehr predict that the flawed random family either collapses to an authoritarian closed family, outside authorities intervene, or the chaos continues until the random family is emotionally if not physically torn apart (1975).

When faced with crisis, the open family tends to overwhelm itself with too much information, too many people, and endless discussions. Their core purpose of adaptation through consensus places family members in a double bind (Kantor & Lehr, 1975, pp. 153–154): "We must resolve this crisis, yet we need more information before we can decide anything." The open family's quest for "emotional authenticity" leads to a "burlesque of exuberance" or "members either withdraw emotionally . . . or physically leave . . . by separations and divorces. . . . " (Kantor & Lehr, 1975, p. 155).

DIVORCE TRAJECTORIES

A divorce trajectory for each family type starts with a summary of Kantor and Lehr's description of each family's usual patterns of functioning followed by an elaboration of plausible antecedents and responses to divorce for each family. These divorce trajectories by no means cover all problems and solutions. Instead, they illustrate vulnerabilities and strengths which are consistent with each family type's values.

A Closed Family: Coping with Divorce as Disaster

According to Kantor and Lehr (1975), in their usual routine, the McKenzie family works together like a simple well-oiled machine. Mom and Dad are unquestionably in charge with Dad as the undisputed "chief" and Mom as "second in command." The seven children, ages 4 to 14, are better acquainted with their parents as a couple, the parental authority, than as individuals. John, the eldest child, has some authority over his younger siblings, but he also must set a good example for them. Discipline is rigorously enforced and is seen as essential training for achievement in the outside world, beginning with excellence in school work and local sports events.

The McKenzies' expression of affect and access to intimacy is firmly regulated. Strong emotions are rarely expressed in public or in the home. Even seeking affection at best is discouraged and at worse is put down or punished. Open fighting is prohibited. Outside visitors are few in number and carefully screened. All family members' comings and goings are closely monitored (Kantor & Lehr, 1975).

What might lead this serene, tight-knit family to divorce? A major disruption to their sense of tradition and order could trigger a divorce. Consider the following scenario. Trouble starts for the family when Mr. McKenzie loses his job and is unable to find employment. Mrs. McKenzie finds work as a waitress, while Mr. McKenzie stays home with the children. Because of their preference for tradition and stability, all the family members experience difficulty with these changes. Mother hates working outside the home; she feels guilty about neglecting her role as mother and homemaker (Mortimer & London, 1984). Dad feels "unmanned" without his traditional role as "breadwinner" (Komarovski, 1940). The children are confused and upset by Dad's sullen presence at home and Mom's irritability after work, yet the family prohibitions on expression of affect permit little discussion about these changes. Dad and Mom's usual partnership has been disrupted by their role reversal, neither feels confident to enforce discipline on his or her own, and the children become lax in doing their chores. The parents alternate between feeling inadequate to correct the children and ignoring their lapses or overreacting with harsh punishment. They then quarrel about who is being too lenient or too strict.

Unsuccessful attempts to enforce traditional rules and maintain emotional calm in a nontraditional, confusing situation convince the McKenzies that their family life is intolerable. Mr. McKenzie has an affair with one of the neighbor women, who has been helping him with the housework and children. When Mrs. McKenzie discovers the affair, she is outraged. Not only is she doing her husband's job when she would rather be home with the children, she feels betrayed by the partner she trusted. The children also feel betrayed, ally with Mom, and help her evict Dad the day the affair is discovered without deliberation or discussion. Mrs. McKenzie files for divorce. Neither Mr. McKenzie nor the children question her actions.

In spite of the McKenzies' belief that divorce is inevitable under the circumstances, the following months are painful, confusing, and difficult for all members of the family. The McKenzies are caught in a paradox: they must be a family, yet the affair represents the ultimate breach of family loyalty. Also, the McKenzies have no tradition for dealing with divorce.

How might this closed family adapt to divorce? In view of their preference for traditional roles and dislike for change, two possibilities seem likely. One is relatively rapid remarriage, e.g., Mr. McKenzie might remarry, have more children, and thus duplicate the closed family system he prefers. Another possibility is dependence on extended family members, e.g., Mrs. McKenzie might recruit an "insider" such as her brother or father as an adult partner to ease her role strain as a single parent. A third possibility would be elevation of the eldest son to the role of "man of the house." Continued contact between ex-spouses seems unlikely in view of Mr. McKenzie's perceived breach of loyalty which has thrust him outside the family's membership.

These two new closed families may reflect adequate postdivorce adaptations for the MacKenzies. However, Mr. MacKenzie may not find a new wife who shares his values, or Mrs. MacKenzie may not have a suitable relative to help her raise the family. The eldest son is at risk to becoming "parentified," i.e., overinvolved in adult concerns and resented by his younger siblings. Also, old issues, i.e., the estrangement between the children and their father, and future disruptions to their stability, i.e., changes in finances and maturation of the children, could lead to new crises. Specifically, dating, sexuality, and leaving home are often troublesome for closed families, because these changes challenge existing rules, roles, and boundaries.

The author worked with a closed Irish-American family in which similar issues were highly problematic. The identified client, 17, had been arrested for stealing and had impregnated his 16-year-old girl friend. Another son, 21, was experimenting with homosexuality. A daughter, 20, had been offered an out-of-state summer job, but her parents wanted her to stay home. Disagreements over management of the children were straining the parents' marriage. This family was caught in a closed-family paradox of wanting its members to be independent, competent, and disciplined, yet as the children approached adulthood, they were not permitted to leave home. Apparently, the only way to independence was to do something sufficiently terrible to be "thrown out of the house" (e.g., become delinquent or homosexual). This case suggests problems which could loom ahead for the McKenzies as their children mature.

An Open Family: Divorce as Adaptation

According to Kantor and Lehr (1975), the Cloud family has always prided themselves in their "openness": honest, genuine expression of all kinds of emotions, tolerance and discussion of all sorts of ideas, the number and diversity of friends and visitors who feel free to stop in any time, and, most of all, their ability to make decisions and solve problems democratically. As an architect, Mr. Cloud sees many clients at his office in the family home. As a therapist, Mrs. Cloud spends long hours seeing clients outside the home. The children, Peter, 12, and Susanna, 9, often have friends over for dinner and to spend the night. Finding sufficient time to pursue activities as individuals, as a family, and with friends is a constant challenge (Kantor & Lehr, 1975).

What would lead this friendly, democratic family to divorce? Here is one possible scenario. After extensive family discussions, the Clouds decide to have an open marriage. Though open marriage generated strong emotions and heated discussions, the Clouds do not view it as the "cause" of their divorce (Constantine, 1984). Nor do the Clouds see "role reversal" (e.g., Mr. Cloud's being home with the children more than Mrs. Cloud) as causing their divorce. Instead, they are proud of their liberated roles and relationships. Factors leading to the divorce include the more general issues of too little time to pursue all their individual and joint interests, too little energy to discuss and decide everything openly and fairly, and too little privacy due to the constant stream of friends and visitors (Constantine, 1983, 1984).

Though Mr. and Mrs. Cloud initially felt their open marriage enhanced their own intimacy and sexual interest, the "care and feeding" of extramarital relationships has become another demand on time and energy, another issue to discuss and decide with the family. The lovers exert additional demands and pressure. Mrs. Cloud's lover wants her to leave her husband. Mr. Cloud's lover initially found his family's openness intriguing, but she soon found the endless negotiations and infrequent opportunities to be alone with Mr. Cloud unacceptable. She broke off the relationship. Mr. Cloud finds his pangs of jealousy and rejection embarrassingly contrary to his open values, but the pangs are undeniable and uncomfortable.

The Clouds discuss everything, yet it seems that nothing gets decided. Mr. Cloud is missing deadlines for his clients; his architecture business has fallen off sharply. Mrs. Cloud is feeling increasingly drained and ineffective as a therapist. In efforts to claim more of their parents' attention, the children have been more obstreperous; this behavior in turn stimulates further family discussions.

Out of frustration and exhaustion, Mrs. Cloud moves out into a friend's apartment. The family is upset. They have always been proud of their tolerance and ability to negotiate all sort of problems. Mr. Cloud and the children alternate between anger at each other and the absent Mrs. Cloud, and crying and comforting each other. Mrs. Cloud stays up all night talking to her friend then sleeps for two days straight.

After a few weeks, the situation, at least on the surface, does not seem very different. Mrs. Cloud often visits the rest of the family. Everyone voraciously reads books about creative divorce, divorce mediation, joint custody and pumps divorced friends for information. Family members see various therapists. Discussions about whether to divorce continue off and on for several years. Though the indecision seems unbearable at times, the Clouds keep finding new issues and information to discuss.

Eventually, Mr. and Mrs. Cloud find new intimate partners. Both feel less pressure to discuss and express their feelings to each other as their lives move apart. The decision to divorce seems natural and desirable. Yet, the Clouds are still good friends and see each other often. They work out an elaborate split-week joint-custody arrangement for the children. Naturally, Peter and Susanna are included in discussions about where they want to live, with whom, and how much of the time. Mr. Cloud marries his new partner; she and her three children from her previous marriage move into the house. Mrs. Cloud finds an apartment of her own, keeps in touch with many of their common friends, and dates several men. Keeping in touch while adding more people to their family network is consistent with the Clouds' open values.

This enlarged open family may function adequately for the Clouds, but it has several vulnerabilities. A sudden change may require a quick decision, a difficult task for the Clouds, given their penchant for sharing feelings, information-gathering, and negotiation. Less articulate family members, particularly children, may feel overburdened by expectations that they articulate their feelings and views and share responsibility in decision-making (Constantine, 1983). Children may feel ignored amidst adult pursuits of complex relationships and multiple interests and may either act out or retreat into depression or thoughts of suicide. Or "warring factions" may form, perhaps between the two sets of children (i.e., Peter/Susanna and their step siblings).

In a therapeutic consultation (Whitaker, 1985), the author observed a large, tribe-like open family whose members seemed isolated, angry, and confused. The "tribe" consisted of a therapist, his third wife, their new baby, their assorted children from previous marriages including an adult divorced daughter and her children, and their therapist who was also a business associate and friend of the family. Family members used fashionable jargon about sharing, intimacy, and bonding, but they appeared to be detached from one another. The marriage was in serious trouble. The patriarch, who ran weekend encounter groups in their home, appeared remote and emotionally burned out. His new wife described herself as lacking self-esteem and overwhelmed by all the children and the expectation that she cook for the large household as well as weekend encounter guests. The adult daughter appeared to be angry and jealous of the new wife. The children looked lost, like waifs left to fend for themselves. Their therapist expressed confusion about her role, including whose friend or therapist she was. This family exhibited many of the symptoms of the emotional exhaustion, confused roles, and blurred boundaries which characterize dysfunctional open families (Kantor & Lehr, 1975; Constantine, 1983, 1984). This case suggests some of the potential difficulties which could face the Clouds.

A Random Family: Divorce as a Creative Paradox

According to Kantor and Lehr, the Canwin family experiences a creative chaos which both delights and frustrates them. There are no set rules except that individual choice usually has priority over collective family goals, but there is ambiguity even on this point. The Canwin's mealtime dilemma epitomizes the contradictions inherent in their random lifestyle. All four family members individually decry the fact that mealtimes do not provide opportunities for more sharing and closeness. Yet, to set aside a specific time of day and require all members to be present violates each person's right to be elsewhere, doing what s/he wants to do, when s/he wants to do it. Closeness and intimacy do occur, but emotional exchanges are not only unplanned but also unpredictable in both intensity and range. Son Teddy, 9, affectionately insults his mother and shouts epithets at his father. Daughter Melissa, 13, is free to compete openly with her mother for her father's physical affection. Though

Mrs. Canwin is the most avid defender of individual freedoms, she is usually the one to call a halt to chaos, even when she herself is enjoying the whimsy and paradox.

Dad occasionally acknowledges his personal preference for more traditional arrangements, such as more parental control, regular mealtimes, and greater respect for personal privacy and possessions, but he usually accedes to the family preference for the random style of interaction. However, his occasional authoritarian harangues cause considerable confusion and uncertainty both to himself and to other family members. Teddy has put a lock on his bedroom door to prevent the others from using his clothes or toys (Kantor & Lehr, 1975).

What would lead this delightful cast of zany characters to divorce? Each family member probably would have their own "divorce story." Teddy claims the divorce started when Melissa started picking the lock on his door and messing around with his computer games. Teddy was enraged; he used a more complicated lock, but she decoded that one too. Mr. Canwin criticized Melissa for infringing Teddy's privacy, while Mrs. Canwin praised Melissa's resourcefulness. Mr. Canwin claims the divorce goes back to his disagreement with his wife about how to handle Teddy. After the lock incident, Teddy began to withdraw, create an elaborate secret language, and talk to invisible companions. Mrs. Canwin respected his behavior as "creative," but Mr. Canwin wanted him examined by a psychiatrist. Melissa claims the divorce started when Mr. Canwin took Teddy to a therapist. A huge fight followed, which escalated into violence. The neighbors called the police. Both Mr. and Mrs. Canwin required stitches; the children, who jumped into the fray, suffered cuts and bruises. The hysteria and drama continued at the hospital emergency room; between police questioning, medical examination and treatment of various family members, the Canwins could not decide who should file charges against whom. Mr. Canwin and Teddy left the hospital and went to a motel instead of returning home, which Mrs. Canwin considered the beginning of the divorce.

After several months of stormy arguments, reconciliations, and separations, the Canwins legally divorced. However, they continue to sleep together, argue over how to manage Teddy, and enjoy outrageously good times. Without openly discussing it, the Canwins have come to a paradoxical arrangement: they are divorced yet together. In this arrangement, Mr. Canwin feels less overwhelmed and has more conviction to stand up for his views. Without Mr. Canwin and Teddy in the house to temper their exuberance, mother and daughter have had to temper themselves. Teddy also has benefitted from a less chaotic environment. His secret languages and invisible companions now resemble the games of an imaginative 9-year-old rather than a desperate retreat from invasive disorder. Frequent visits from separate homes seem to strike a workable balance between destructive and creative chaos for the Canwins.

Though this account ends on a positive upswing, the Canwins are at risk for future random family vulnerabilities. The Canwins may miss the chaos of living together. Or chaos may overtake them again in their separate-yet-together arrangement. Their paradoxical arrangement may have initial appeal, but in true random family form, the Canwins may quickly tire of it, even if it is working, in favor of "something new" (Kantor & Lehr, 1975, p. 156). Additionally, lack of support from extended family, friends, and society for their novel postdivorce arrangement could make the Canwins more vulnerable to future difficulties.

In summary, this discussion does not cover all possibilities for each family type. Divorce is not disastrous to all closed families, adaptive to all open families, or creatively paradoxical to all random families. However, these "trajectories" suggest plausible examples of different families' divorce experiences, tapping the potential for both resourcefulness and dysfunction for each family type.

IMPLICATIONS FOR THE THERAPIST

As the preceding divorce trajectories suggest, families can experience and interpret divorce very differently; they may attribute their divorce to diverse causes and respond to divorce in varying ways. Several investigators (Boss & Greenberg, 1984; Hill, 1959) have pointed out the importance of the meaning that families may ascribe to events or circumstances. Others (Pollner & Wikler, 1985; Reiss, 1981) suggest that every family constructs its own "reality" about itself and the world which the family conserves through interactional patterns. Kantor and Lehr do not explicitly discuss meaning and constructed reality in this sense, but these ideas are implicit in statements such as "what feels like coercion to the open- or random-type systems feels like a natural necessity in the closed system" (1975, p. 146). In this discussion employment and extra-familial relationships serve as examples of issues which can have widely differing meanings for different family types with respect to divorce. For example, the McKenzies saw role reversal and the affair as causes of their divorce. In contrast, the Clouds did not view divorce as a negative consequence of extramarital relationships and role reversal; instead, divorce was seen as a positive adaptation to their liberated roles and relationships. Whereas the McKenzies generated two new, separate closed families, the Clouds expanded their family boundaries to include new partners and step-children. In the Canwin's case, extra-marital affairs and role reversal were irrelevant to divorce.

These different meanings for similar events, in this case changes in family-work roles, extramarital affairs, and divorce, suggest several therapeutic implications. In assisting families who are considering, experiencing, or adjusting to divorce, a family therapist can be more effective if she or he has some sense of what divorce means and what responses are acceptable for each family. For example, expecting Mrs. McKenzie to "forgive" her husband's affair might be as unrealistic as expecting Mrs. Cloud to "condemn" her husband's. Similarly, the therapist who is distracted in condemning the Clouds for their open marriage might overlook more crippling problems, such as the family's difficulties in bringing closure to decisions.

Additionally, the three families deal with affect differently. Much therapeutic literature urges freer expression of affect, which often benefits closed families who have difficulty experiencing and expressing emotion. However, emotionally exhausted open families or emotionally overwhelmed random families need less affective expression and more structure conducive to productive decision-making which benefits all family members. For example, the open family may need help to devise a time-limited decision-making strategy to bypass their endless information-gathering and discussion cycle. A therapist might assist the random family develop a means to referee their emotional outbursts.

Like meaning and affect, each family types' sense of time varies. Because the closed family values stability and tends to avoid change or uncertainty, the McKenzies are depicted as coming to a relatively rapid re-establishment of stability, through the creation of two new closed families, perhaps within the year. On the other hand, because the open family values discussion and negotiation, their decision to divorce and postdivorce adaptation could take considerably longer, as in the Clouds' case, several years. The Canwins' erratic sense of time tends to defy prediction. With respect to these different time frames, a therapist who is unaware of the closed family's intolerance for unstability may be skeptical of the family's urgency to re-establish stability in the form of rapid remarriage, dependence on extended family members, or parentification of the oldest child. Indeed, these tactics do not guarantee the stability a closed family wants and in fact have their own risks. However, closed families are more likely to view these tactics as acceptable postdivorce options than open or random families. Similarly, the therapist's impatience with the random family's changeability and the open family's longer time frame may be counterproductive.

Alternatively, the therapist can help each family "create" a meaning for its divorce which could be useful to its members. For example, using the Milan group's concept of positive connotation (Palazzoli-Selvini, Boscolo, Cecchin & Prata, 1978), the therapist could suggest that the McKenzies have used the divorce to express their traditional values of discipline and hard work to build two new families. Similarly, the therapist could remind the Clouds that their divorce has made their family larger and more inclusive, reinforcing their pride in their "open door" policy. The therapist's validation of the Canwin's "separate yet together" divorce as a workable paradox may be an effective confirmation of their random family values in the face of society's skepticism, even antagonism, toward their unusual arrangement.

Hetherington (1981) noted that most research has viewed the divorced family as a pathogenic family and has failed to focus on positive postdivorce functioning. In response to Hetherington's observation and in the spirit of Kantor and Lehr's efforts to present both strengths and weaknesses of three family types, this discussion depicts plausible adaptations and vulnerabilities for each family's hypothetical divorce. Additionally, the three families' different divorce trajectories suggest that the "divorce process" may vary considerably from family to family. Consideration of divorce trajectories for Kantor and Lehr's three family types suggests two new research avenues. First, in statistical terms, "family type" as a variable may account for a significant amount of variance in the "causes," "effects," and "processes" of divorce. Needless to say, operationalization of family type poses difficult research problems. Alternately, the divorce trajectories for Kantor and Lehr's family types provide a qualitative overview of the complexity of divorce and ways it can vary from family to family. Finally, consideration of divorce in terms family interaction complements sociological research on demographic differences and psychological research on the individual who experiences divorce.

NOTES

1. While a critique of Kantor and Lehr's work is beyond the scope of this discussion, a brief note about their definitions of the three family types is in order. First, Kantor and Lehr do not define the term ''family,'' but their discussion emphasizes nuclear intact families. Second, Kantor and Lehr's theoretical definitions of the three family types, with their myriad variables and neologisms, are problematic; they confuse rather than clarify family differences. However, the case sketches make each family type come alive. Thus, this discussion emphasizes Kantor and Lehr's case sketches.

2. Kantor and Lehr note that their three family types rarely exist in their ''pure'' forms. Instead, most families are a mixture of these types. For example, a particular family may be open in its expression of affect, closed in its power structure, and random in its value of creativity and paradox. Also, Constantine (1983, 1984) has suggested that families can evolve from one type to another. However, the three ''pure'' types represent a heuristic simplification against which real families can be compared. For the sake of brevity, this discussion is confined to the three pure types.

3. Kantor and Lehr's (1975) suggestion that the emergence of a flawed family type is ''symptomatic'' of a family experiencing crisis implies a unidirectional relationship between crisis and flawed types, i.e., crisis causes a flawed family type. There are two problems with this implication. First, the relationshp between crises and family dysfunction seems likely to be biodirectional. Not only can crises contribute to family dysfunction but also dysfunctional families create crises for themselves and for larger systems (i.e., educational, legal, health care systems). Second, the term ''flawed type'' does not do justice to Kantor and Lehr's notion that all three family types can be either functional or dysfunctional. The term ''flawed type'' connotes a permanent, unchanging state or fate of dysfunction rather than dysfunction which may be temporary or treatable.

REFERENCES

Boss, P. & Greenberg, J. (1984). Family boundary ambiguity: A new variable in family stress theory. *Family Process*, 23, 535–546.

Caplan, G. (1964). *Principles of Preventative Psychiatry*. New York: Basic Books, Inc.

Constantine, L. L. (1983). Dysfunction and failure in open family systems, I: Application of a unified theory. *Journal of Marriage and the Family*, 45, 725–738.

Constantine, L. L. (1984). Dysfunction and failure in open family systems, II: Clinical issues. *Journal of Marital and Family Therapy*, 10, 1–17.

Erickson, E. H. (1959). Identity and the life cycle. *Psychological Issues*. 1(1).

Hetherington, E. M. (1981). Children and divorce. *Parent-Child Interaction: Theory, Research, and Prospects*. New York: Academic Press, Inc.

Hill, R. (1958). Generic features of families under stress. *Social Casework*, 39, 139–150.

Kantor, D. & Lehr, W. (1975). *Inside the Family*, New York: Harper Colophon Books.

Komarovski, M. (1940). *The Unemployed Man And His Family*. New York: Dryden.

Kraus, S. (1979). The crisis of divorce: Growth promoting or pathogenic? *Journal of Divorce*, 3, 107–119.

Mortimer, J. T. & London, J. (1984). The varying linkages of work and family. In P. Voydanoff (Ed.) *Work and Family*. Palo Alto: Mayfield Publishing Company.

Palazzoli-Selvini, M., Boscolo, L., Ceccin, G. & Prata, G. (1978). *Paradox and Counterparadox: A New Model in the Therapy of the Family in Schizophrenic Transaction*. New York: Jason Aronson.

Pollner, M. & Wikler, L. (1985). The social construction of unreality. *Family Process*, 24, 241–253.

Reiss, D. (1981). *The Family's Construction of Reality*, Cambridge: Harvard University Press.

Watzlawick, P. Weakland, J. H. & Fisch, R. (1974). *Change*. New York: W. W. Norton & Company.

Whitaker, C. (1985). Family therapy consultation/demonstration interview. University of Connecticut Health Center, Department of Psychiatry, Farmington, Connecticut.

DYSFUNCTIONAL MARITAL PATTERNS

The Ambivalent Spouse Syndrome

Bruce William Jones

ABSTRACT. This paper describes some common characteristics of 13 cases in which one marital partner initiated therapy because the other partner was undecided about continuing their marriage. The initiating clients wanted their marriages to continue even if they were unrewarding. They resisted change and denied that change might be taking place. They saw themselves as helpless victims. They were passive, non-assertive, dependent, enmeshed, and had low self-esteem. Those clients who made the most dramatic changes were those who could turn their attention from the ambivalent spouse to their own growth.

A couple experiencing marital difficulty will frequently consult a marriage therapist, either for help in strengthening their relationship or to discuss whether or not they want to end their marriage. Sometimes one partner comes to therapy alone, although increasingly therapists are insisting on seeing the couple together. This paper describes a particular variation on this common theme, in which one partner initiates treatment specifically because the other spouse is uncertain about continuing the marriage. The partner who initiates therapy wants the relationship to continue, even if

Bruce William Jones, PhD, is a Marriage, Family, and Child Counselor in private practice, and Professor at California State College, Bakersfield, P.O. Box 9501, Bakersfield, CA 93389.

Acknowledgement is made to California Family Study Center, Burbank, California, where the clients described in this paper were treated.

it is an unrewarding one. This initiating client usually comes alone, looking for support and for help in maintaining the marriage. When the ambivalent spouse does participate, he or she may miss sessions, participate passively, or drop out altogether. More active participation carries the risk that the marriage might be strengthened.

The initiating clients are not asking for growth or change in self. Their presenting problem is that their spouses are ambivalent. They see themselves as helpless victims. They either do not know what they want from therapy or they want something the therapist cannot provide, that is, to motivate their spouses to be enthusiastic about their marriages. Usually the only personal problems these clients acknowledge are depression and feelings of powerlessness, for which they blame their spouses. In fact, they often suffer from low self-esteem, which predisposes them to tolerate mistreatment from the ambivalent spouses because they fear (1) that they deserve it or (2) that they can do no better. They do not assert themselves with their ambivalent spouses for fear of losing them. They do not admit that they may have already lost them.

LITERATURE REVIEW

Many writers have discussed the relationship between marital quality and marital stability. Marriages that appear happy may end in divorce, whereas unhappy ones may endure (Lenthall, 1977). Dissatisfied couples may disengage emotionally but remain together in a "marriage of convenience" (Lyons, 1979). Others may actually be on a path leading to eventual divorce if one partner has passed the "psychological point of no return," consciously or unconsciously (Frederico, 1979). The quality of a marriage may be the most important determinant of whether it will continue, but stability is also influenced negatively by the attraction to alternatives and positively by barriers to divorce or pressures to remain married (Green & Sporakowski, 1983; Kalb, 1983; Levinger, 1976; Lewis & Spanier, 1979; Spanier & Lewis, 1980, 1981; Thibaut & Kelley, 1959; Thompson & Spanier, 1983).

The decision to divorce or not may be explained in terms of exchange theory, the balance between costs and rewards (Kitson, Holmes, & Sussman, 1983). Dissatisfied couples will remain married if they think that the alternatives available to them are more negative (Albrecht, Bahr, & Goodman, 1983; Albrecht & Kunz, 1980). This seems to be especially true for persons with low self-esteem (Kitson, 1982; Lazarus, 1981).

Sharpe (1981) has described the "symbiotic marriage" in which a couple is so fused that neither partner can function autonomously. They fear being alone. When one partner comes alone to therapy, he or she "invariably has an urgent need to talk almost exclusively about the other one" (Sharpe, 1981, p. 99). When enmeshed couples consider divorce, they remain highly ambivalent and are unprepared to let go of the relationship (Kressel, Jaffee, Tuchman, Watson, & Deutsch, 1980). When they do divorce, persons who have strong attachment to their spouses experience greater distress in separating (Brown, Felton, Whiteman, & Manela, 1980; White & Bloom, 1981). Those who are least likely to adjust well to divorce are submissive, insecure, shy and dependent (Thomas, 1982). Dependent, traditional women who are more concerned to please their husbands than themselves are especially vulnerable (Bloom & Clement, 1984).

Kessler (1975, p. 78) noted that the anticipation of a divorce is often more devastating than the reality. Weiss (1975, 1976) has described the way that the thought of separation frightens some married persons. He compares their attachment to a spouse with a battered child's attachment to his or her parents. Even when the child is mistreated, it wants to return to its parents, "because they are the only parents it has" (Weiss, 1975, p. 97; 1976, p. 137).

When one spouse wants a divorce, the partner who is left may deny the reality to self or others (Ibrahim, 1984; Kressel et al., 1980; Weiss, 1975). Wiseman (1975) has said that both spouses experience a form of emotional crisis in the divorce process, including denial, ambivalence, anger, and depression. In the particular form of that crisis described in this paper one partner appears to express the emotional pain and depression on behalf of both, while the other spouse acts out the ambivalence for both. Both may be involved in denial.

THE SYNDROME

The following description is presented with the belief that there are certain common features—a syndrome—in such cases, and that it is helpful to the therapist to be aware of them. The description is based upon 13 cases from Los Angeles County treated by the author. They participated in therapy for a mean of 10.5 sessions. Divorce proceedings had begun prior to treatment in three cases. Therapy was initiated by the husband in five cases and by the wife in eight cases. The initiating clients varied in age from 28 to 64 with a mean of 40. In five cases, the spouse participated in therapy, but four of those five spouses terminated before the initiating client. Two of the spouses used conjoint sessions to announce in the presence of the therapist that they had decided on divorce. This suggests that the spouse is not always as ambivalent as the initiating client wants to believe. At least eight of the spouses had already found new partners by the time therapy began.

The phrase "ambivalent spouse syndrome" does not mean that the initiating client is ambivalent about *being* a spouse, but rather than he or she *has* an ambivalent spouse. The syndrome consists of being told by one's spouse that he or she has not decided whether to remain married. It is characterized by the features described above: denial, low self-esteem, dependence, enmeshment in a symbiotic relationship, passivity, lack of assertiveness, depression, feeling like a victim, fear of change. These characteristics will be illustrated by referring to the 13 cases.

Denial

Denial was common among the initiating clients in one form or another. One had been separated for six months at his wife's request, while she decided whether to divorce, reconcile, or remain separated. All during that time, he maintained a facade of marriage, telling only one or two close friends of the separation. Another client was convinced that her husband had not been unfaithful to her, even after his new female friend had moved into his house with him.

A 52-year-old woman, married 23 years, illustrates the reluctance of these clients to admit that their marriages might be over. She and her husband had lived separately for seven years, sometimes 2,000 miles apart. Neither partner had been interested in a divorce during that time. The woman did not seek therapy until her husband's ambivalence turned into a desire for divorce, when she became extremely depressed. She hoped that counseling would help to win him back.

Low Self-Esteem

During their seven years of separation, this client's husband had shown little interest in her, except to borrow money from her, but she continued to speak of ways she "had failed" him. She had been born when her mother was 14 years old, and she said she was "begrudgingly" raised by her maternal grandmother. She reported that her husband was the only person who ever gave her any love, so she was reluctant to "let go" of him, even though he had not shown any of that love for seven years. The client was an attractive woman and was very successful financially and professionally, becoming a partner in her company, but she did not believe herself to be worthy of a relationship with a man.

The clients in this group who seemed to be the most resistant to change or to assert themselves with their mates were those who had come to believe that they did not deserve much affection. They had learned to cling desperately to what little they did receive. One reported having intercourse with the spouse about 30 times in 12 years, another about 50 times in 18 years. The husband of another refused to talk to her, though they continued to coexist in the same house. This latter client said she was not aware of any anger toward her husband, though he made no attempt to hide the fact that he was dating other women. She said, rather, "I feel guilty for not giving him everything." Each of these clients preferred to remain married rather than give up what little affection they had. Ten of the clients described here had little support system apart from the ambivalent spouse. Even if the spouse did not give much support, he or she was better than nothing in the eyes of the client.

Enmeshment

The enmeshment of the couples in this report is indicated by the fact that the ambivalent spouse, like the initiating client, was often unable to break away from the marriage, no matter how unsatisfying he or she considered it to be. Both partners seemed quite dependent. One couple had separated briefly eight years previously, but had seen each other every day during the separation. This ambivalent wife left home twice during the course of therapy, but never stayed away more than one night. In conjoint sessions she talked about how unhappy she was being married, but she remained. The husband, likewise, complained about her, but resisted any change. Even though the wife had affairs with the knowledge of her husband, he feared that if he objected to them, she would carry out her threat to leave him.

Non-Assertiveness

One of the most obvious features of such persons is that they appear passive. At the beginning of therapy, 12 out of the 13 initiating clients were unwilling to assert themselves with their spouses. Although eight of the spouses were engaged in outside relationships, only one client explicitly asked her husband to end an affair with another woman. If the ambivalent spouses did not move out while making up their minds, in all cases but one they were permitted to stay by their mates. The one exception—the same woman who asked her husband to end his affair—eventually asked her husband to leave after discussing that decision in several sessions of therapy and after changing her mind frequently. One client of the 13 voluntarily moved out of her own residence, not in anger, she said, but in the hope that, by making no demands upon her husband, he would choose to ask her back.

Lack of Power

Some of the clients were quite successful in their careers, but saw themselves as helpless in their marriages. Not surprisingly, they were quite depressed. All but one of the initiating clients saw themselves as helpless victims at the beginning of treatment. They wanted something only their spouses could provide. The old truism applies here: The one who cares least about a relationship has the most power in it.

The spouse's ambivalence, of course, is a way of exercising the ultimate power: to decide whether the marriage lives or dies. One couple came to therapy together at the urging of the 64-year-old husband. They had separated, by the wife's decision, and she had begun divorce proceedings, but she was still ambivalent to the extent that she agreed to delay further action. She consented to accompany her husband to therapy provided that he pay for it with his separate funds. What she really wanted, she said, was individual therapy to work on her own growth. The financial arrangements for therapy were indicative of their balance of power at that time. She complained that her husband had been "controlling" during their years together, but she was able to take control of their relationship by beginning a divorce her husband did not want and then delaying it. She would agree to see her husband occasionally, but only on her terms.

Fear of Change

One client who insisted strongly that her husband would not come to conjoint therapy admitted later that she did not want him to come because she feared he would resolve his indecision by ending their marriage. She explained that she would rather have "half an apple" than none at all. This client's husband, just turned 40, had an affair with a younger woman, and moved 90 miles away from his wife to take another job. He visited her and their two children every weekend. He would alternately tell her that he did and did not love her. He would make love with her on some occasions and talk about divorce on others. She reported his vague references to future plans for the two of them and then asked, pleadingly, "That doesn't sound like he wants a divorce, does it?"

This client said that her husband had all the power in their relationship, including the power to end it. She had little support system apart from her husband, and she feared losing him. Occasionally she would ask him to leave, but would always change her mind. Like the partners in a symbiotic marriage, she consistently wanted to talk about her husband in each session rather than about herself. The therapist could see little difference in her between her first and her last (eighth) session. The therapist explained that he could not change her absent husband, and asked what her goals were in counseling. "To cope," she said, "so that nothing will need to change."

TREATMENT

The implicit goal of the initiating clients was to prevent change or to restore a status quo. Some of them, however, recognized that that was either impossible in their situations or undesirable. These clients moved from being helpless and depressed to planning for change. They learned to focus on themselves, either on changes they wanted to make, their own self-esteem, their own patterns in relationships, or their families of origin. Those who made no resolution continued to talk primarily about the ambivalent spouse and what he or she wanted.

For some clients, change came quickly, for others slowly. One had a series of 24 sessions over a period of 10 months. Her husband had an affair, said he preferred the new woman, but refused to leave his wife. For a long time, the client's indecision seemed to be as great as her husband's. One week she would decide to seek a legal separation; the next she would want to give the marriage another try. She terminated therapy, saying she had completed her transition and was making a new life; later, she would begin again, wondering whether she should "let go" of the husband who did not want her. Then, at one point, she said that her husband was "not worth worrying about." Subsequently, she began to turn away from complaints about her husband and trying to figure out what he wanted. Then she could examine her own patterns of behavior. Therapy included some productive sessions with her family of origin.

Another client made a comparable transition within the first week. Her husband was living with another woman, but said he did not know what he wanted with regard to his marriage. In her first session, the client showed very low self-esteem. She had been a prostitute and drug addict when she met her husband; she wondered whether she "deserved" her current treatment because she had been unfaithful once during their marriage. In her second session, she began to talk realistically about her options for finances, living arrangements, and long-range career plans. She said, "If (my husband) wants to come back, I am going to insist on some changes."

Another woman made equally dramatic changes in herself over the course of six sessions. Nineteen months before therapy began, her husband moved out, saying he no longer loved her. However, he would not file for divorce. He continued to seek his wife's company, and spoke of their house as his "home." During therapy, the client became increasingly independent. She set limits with members of her family of origin, and described herself as more assertive. In the fourth session, she said that she had regained the power in their marriage; the husband who had left was now afraid of losing her. In the following week, she gave her husband an ultimatum, to either return home within six months or get a divorce. At her last (sixth) session, she said she was glad for their separation because of the personal growth that she had made as a result of it. She described herself as feeling better than at any time in her life and proud of her ability to take care of herself. She said she had learned that she could be happy whether married or single.

Some clients prefer not to make any change. One had agreed to work on her self-esteem and assertiveness, and then she cancelled subsequent appointments. To be more assertive would have upset the uneasy balance that allowed her uncommitted husband to continue under the same roof with her. One man was telling the same stories and making the same complaints about his wife after 26 sessions as he had done in the first session. Sometimes the therapist would be able to encourage him to look at himself and his own role in the marriage, but only briefly. Invariably, he would resume talking about his wife. Complaining about his fate had become his habitual substitute for changing it. Three months after termination he reported that their relationship was basically unchanged.

We have already noted that the fear of divorce may be more devastating than divorce itself. With these clients, the anticipation was incapacitating. When they started to deal with what was happening in their marriages, they were able to make dramatic changes.

DISCUSSION

The characteristics of a particular type of client have been described, based on 13 cases in which clients sought therapy because they said their spouses could not decide between marriage or divorce. It is quite clear that both partners are resisting change. They are comfortable in their discomfort. The initiating spouse does not want the marriage to get worse or to end. The ambivalent spouse does not want it to get better. The therapist is a threat to the uneasy equilibrium of their marital system.

The therapist should take time to help the client decide whether the marriage can be saved. If at all possible, this should be done in conjoint sessions. To the therapist's way of thinking, the marriage may be unworkable, but only the couple has the right to make that judgment. If the spouse has not already made a tacit decision for divorce and really is ambivalent, there is a chance for reconciliation, and conjoint sessions can work toward strengthening the marriage. If the couple is moving toward divorce, then counseling can smooth the way for the separating couple, and the therapist can help the rejected client grieve for his or her loss and plan for the future.

REFERENCES

Albrecht, S. L.; Bahr, H. M.; & Goodman, K. L. *Divorce and remarriage: Problems, adaptations, and adjustments*. Westport, CT: Greenwood, 1983.

Albrecht, S. L., & Kunz, P. R. The decision to divorce: A social exchange perspective. *Journal of Divorce*, 1980, 3, 319–337.

Bloom, B. L., & Clement, C. Marital sex role orientation and adjustment to separation and divorce. *Journal of Divorce*, 1984, 7(3), 87–98.

Brown, P.; Felton, B.; Whiteman, V.; & Manela, R. Attachment and distress following marital separation. *Journal of Divorce*, 1980, 3, 303–317.

Federico, J. The marital termination period of the divorce adjustment process. *Journal of Divorce*, 1979, 3, 93–106.

Green, R. G., & Sporakowski, M. J. The dynamics of divorce: Marital quality, alternative attractions and external pressures. *Journal of Divorce*, 1983, 7(2), 77–88.

Ibrahim, A. I. The process of divorce. *Conciliation Courts Review*, 1984, 22, 81–87.

Kalb, M. The conception of the alternative and the decision to divorce. *American Journal of Psychotherapy*, 1983, 37, 346–356.

Kessler, S. *The American way of divorce: Prescriptions for change*. Chicago: Nelson-Hall, 1975.

Kitson, G. C. Attachment to the spouse in divorce: A scale and its application. *Journal of Marriage and the Family*, 1982, 44, 379–393.

Kitson, G. C.; Holmes, W. M.; & Sussman, M. B. Withdrawing divorce petitions: A predictive test of the exchange model of divorce. *Journal of Divorce*, 1983, 7(1), 51–66.

Kressel, K.; Jaffee, N.; Tuchman, B.; Watson, C.; & Deutsch, M. A typology of divorcing couples: Implications for mediation and the divorce process. *Family Process*, 1980, 19, 101–116.

Lazarus, A. A. Divorce counseling or marriage therapy? A therapeutic option. *Journal of Marital and Family Therapy*, 1981, 7, 15–22.

Lenthall, G. Marital satisfaction and marital stability. *Journal of Marriage and Family Counseling*, 1977, 3(4), 25–32.

Levinger, G. A. A social psychological perspective on marital dissolution. *Journal of Social Issues*, 1976, 32(1), 21–47.

Lewis, R. A. & Spanier, G. B. Theorizing about the quality and stability of marriage. In W. R. Burr, R. Hill, F. I. Nye, & I. L. Reiss (Eds.), *Contemporary theories about the family: Research-based theories* (Vol. 1). New York: Free Press, 1979, 268–294.

Lyons, M. C. Marriage of convenience: An alternative to open marriage or creative divorce. *Family Therapy*, 1979, 6, 161–173.

Sharpe, S. A. The symbiotic marriage: A diagnostic profile. *Bulletin of the Menninger Clinic*, 1981, 45, 89–114.

Spanier, G. B., & Lewis, R. A. Marital quality: A review of the seventies. *Journal of Marriage and the Family*, 1980, 42, 825–839.

Spanier, G. B., & Lewis, R. A. Marital quality and marital stability: A reply. *Journal of Marriage and the Family*, 1981, 43, 782–783.

Thibaut, J. W., & Kelley, H. H. *The Social Psychology of Groups*. New York: Wiley, 1959.

Thomas, S. P. After divorce: Personality factors related to the process of adjustment. *Journal of Divorce*, 1982, 5(3), 19–36.

Thompson, L., & Spanier, G. B. The end of marriage and acceptance of marital termination. *Journal of Marriage and the Family*, 1983, 45, 103–113.

Weiss, R. S. *Marital separation*. New York: Basic Books, 1975.
Weiss, R. S. The emotional impact of marital separation. *Journal of Social Issues*, 1976, 32(1), 135–145.
White, S. W., & Bloom, B. L. Factors related to the adjustment of divorcing men. *Family Relations*, 1981, 30, 349–360.
Wiseman, R. S. Crisis theory and the process of divorce. *Social Casework*, 1975, 56, 205–212.

A Comparison of Men Who Are Divorce Prone with Those Who Are Marriage Phobic

Robert M. Counts
Kelly Reid

In an earlier paper, Counts and Sacks (1986) described three personality profiles of Divorce Prone individuals. In that article Divorce Prone was defined as any individual who had been divorced two or more times. The three personality profiles were (1) The Self Involved Narcissist, (2) The Compliant Depressed, and (3) The Casualties of Life's Vicissitudes. The authors noted that these three types of individuals were quite different psychologically, behaviorally, and prognostically. They found that the Self Involved Narcissists were confident, action oriented, and hard driving. These individuals were usually quite successful in their careers. They were creative, innovative, and at times were reckless. They were the ones to leave the marriage, going directly from one marriage to the next with someone waiting in the wings. The Self Involved Narcissists were quick to end relationships for what seemed to be whimsical reasons.

The Compliant Depressed, on the other hand, had many doubts and fears, were uncertain and indecisive, responding vigorously to any loss or separation. They were not as successful in their careers as the Self Involved Narcissist. Usually they were the ones who were deserted and they recovered slowly from the loss. For them, divorce was extremely painful. Before their first marriage and then between marriages, they often had not dated extensively—they may

Robert M. Counts, MD, and Kelly Reid, MD, are on the faculty of the Family Therapy Program, Department of Psychiatry, New York University Medical Center, School of Medicine, New York, NY, and the Center for Marital and Family Therapy, New York, NY.

be alone without a boy friend or girl friend for long periods of time. In relationships with the opposite sex, they were usually dependent and compliant.

Counts and Sacks found the Casualties of Life's Vicissitudes to be less self centered than the Narcissistic group and less unhappy than the Compliant Depressed. While separations and losses were painful to these individuals, they were not overwhelmed. There was little evidence of a repetitive pattern in their marriages or divorces. They were not promiscuous and they seemed to care about others. Their divorces seemed to be more the result of the complicated circumstances of their life than to personality problems.

In the present article we will compare two Self Involved Narcissistic Divorce Prone individuals with two men we are defining as "Marriage Phobic." These latter individuals were fearful of getting married although they professed a wish to do so—they were heterosexual with no known history of homosexual interests or activities. We also have chosen two individuals as representative of this group who, in fact, did marry—one was briefly married at the age of 32. The second married when he was 40 while in psychotherapy with one of the authors (RMC).

We believe that a comparison of these two groups may reveal some interesting notions about the vicissitudes of marriages and divorce.

CASE STUDIES

Group One: The Divorce Prone

*Case 1**

B.P. is a 61 year old three times married, white male living with a woman 36 years his junior who will probably become his fourth wife. He volunteered as a subject for the study when he learned through mutual friends that we were interviewing individuals who had been divorced two or more times.

He was an only child. His parents were divorced when he was nine years old. "The loss of my father was very hard for me." He had almost no contact with his father until he was 18, then saw a lot of him. His mother was a "very strong person who dominated my

*Case 1 was presented in the paper by Counts and Sacks (1986).

childhood.'' He was sent to boarding school when he was 13 years old and this may have served to dilute her oppressive influence. He said, ''I began to enjoy life and I never wanted to go home'' (and see mother). From early childhood he wet the bed—because of this symptom he was repeatedly rejected by the Armed Forces.

He met his first wife, Betty, when he was 16. She came from a background very similar to his own—they were married when he was 25 and she was 24. He described sex during the early years of their marriage as ''adequate but not great.'' They had three children, a daughter who is now 35, a son 31, and a daughter 28. His first wife might be considered a very conventional choice. This marriage continued for 16 years and ended when he became interested in another woman. After the divorce he maintained rather limited contact with his children. His first wife never remarried.

He met Mary, his second wife, when still married to his first. He states, ''We were playing out a romantic love affair—a dream.'' They lived together for three years. As soon as his divorce from Betty (his first wife) was final, they married. Their union lasted for seven years and was childless. His impulsive running off with another woman heralded the end of this relationship. At Mary's suggestion they saw a marital therapist. They did so but the therapist seemed to believe that the relationship with Mary could not be resurrected as he had already been living with Susan for a month. He accepted this verdict without protest and said, ''With Mary (his second wife) the relationship was sufficiently complicated and problematic and I knew it couldn't work if there was an involvement with another woman.'' He seemed to believe that once he had moved on there was no going back. He is still on good terms with Mary and views her as his best friend.

He had met his third wife, Susan, while doing bibliographical research. ''I think she decided she wanted me.'' He said, in speaking of Susan, ''I think I'm a man with repeated behavior. I was repeating the same behavior over and over again.'' This marriage, in contrast to the first two, was very tumultuous. They fought repeatedly from the beginning of the marriage. He was troubled, frightened and depressed by the financial ruin this marriage brought on him. As a result of the emotional turmoil, he briefly sought professional help. He believed that the involvement with Susan was self destructive from beginning to end, although sex was good. This marriage lasted four years, was childless, and he again had someone waiting in the wings.

He had been living with Alice for four years at the time of the interview. She was 36 years his junior. This relationship was reported by him as tranquil and not obviously troubled.

Mr. P. describes himself as a chronic "womanizer." He said, "I think it was a romantic wanting to be in love with someone who had the same romantic feelings toward me as I had toward her." He stated he very much enjoyed repeating this type of experience and the uniqueness of the woman wasn't all that important. After a time he tired of each woman. When asked what would cause him to set out in the pursuit of a new woman, he said, "When my sexual needs struck me strongly enough I would pursue the woman and I was usually successful." He went on to say, "I've wondered if my wetting the bed reduced my self esteem and that I compensated with sex—it was an ego drive."

Mr. P. was not especially upset as a consequence of his three divorces. He had little overt grief and did not seem troubled by guilt. Perhaps these relationships were so superficial and his involvement so tenuous that he experienced no sense of loss. He also felt that his decision to leave was, on each occasion, justified. He protected himself by always being the one to end the relationship. His third marriage and divorce were more stressful than the first two as his wife fought with him and, in the end, was quite vindictive. He was much relieved when it was all over.

Mr. P. seems very self centered, expects a lot from women, and has little to give them. He is handsome, aggressive, articulate, and gifted with much charm. It was easy to see how he had induced many women to do his bidding. In each instance he ended the marriage and then moved to the next. He never had lived alone. He seemed to take little responsibility for his actions and seemed to be saying, "I had no choice. My feelings made me do it."

We believe that the early desertion by his father had sensitized him to loss and then resulted in his entering into relationships tenatively and without a full commitment to the person. Negative feelings such as boredom, anger, or a fear of loss would trigger a quick withdrawal from a relationship to which he had only tentatively and partially committed himself. His subsequent placement in boarding school may also have further crystallized this pattern.

Case 2

D.B. is a 33 year old white male bank loan officer, who was in his second marriage at the time of the initial consultation. He and his wife initially came as a couple. Later they separated when Mr. B. became involved with another woman and announced plans for a third marriage.

Consultation was initiated by Mrs. B. after Mr. B. unexpectedly announced in their seventh year of marriage, that he had not been sexually attracted to her for 6-1/2 years. The subject of Mr. B.'s sexual dissatisfaction had never been brought up during their marriage. Moreover, they had an active sex life. Mrs. B. was very perplexed at Mr. B.'s announcement because they often had agreed that their marriage was ideal. They never fought, compromising quickly whenever a disagreement arose. Mrs. B. had initiated the contact with the hope that Mr. B.'s dissatisfaction would be explored and then resolved.

Mr. B. was the oldest of two, with a sister four years his junior. Mr. B.'s parents divorced when he was 17. He said that he had previously believed his parents had a happy and stable marriage. Thus, he was shocked to hear of their plans. Their divorce made him feel that he lacked the ability to tell when a relationship was good and when it wasn't. He never directly connected that feeling to the difficulties he had in his own marriages. His father had initiated the end of the relationship, although Mr. B. felt that his mother also believed this was necessary. Nonetheless, he remembers his mother being emotionally devastated at that time. He sided with her and made, what he later described as, an awkward attempt to comfort her.

Mr. B. said that he had always been uncomfortable around women, feeling that he went unnoticed by them. He said that relationships never progressed to the level of physical involvement. This became a consistent hurdle which he felt he'd never overcome. His first marriage lasted less than a year, and had begun while he was still in college. He states his first wife encouraged his sexual advances, otherwise they would never have gotten involved. He entered into marriage at the prompting of his mother, who wished the couple would get out of the house, as they had taken up permanent residence in her home. He recalls feeling indifferent to the issue of marriage initially, although he thought it was the most logical course of action. By the wedding day, he recalls feeling that he was doing the wrong thing, and wondering why he was taking this step. Nonetheless, they married. After one year of what he describes as a bland relationship, he requested that they separate. His wife was agreeable to this course of action.

Mr. B. continued to have the same problems in single life that he had prior to his first marriage. He saw himself as unattractive to women. He met his second wife at a bus stop. They began to date and were soon involved sexually. They married six months after their first meeting. Mr. B. says that even at the time of their marriage, he felt that "she wasn't the image of the type of woman I could imagine myself with." This "image" apparently remained in his mind thoughout their marriage and was associated with his growing dissatisfaction.

Shortly after marriage, Mr. and Mrs. B. took a trip to Asia. He was impressed with the beauty of Oriental women. He also felt that they, in contrast to American women, noticed him. He found this attention a new and pleasant experience. Following that trip he decided that one day he would return to Asia, with or without his wife, and live there permanently. To that end, he entered the world of banking and finance. His wife put off finishing her undergraduate education to work and help pay for his graduate school expenses. She knew of his interest in international finance, his intrigue with the Far East, and his desire to some day work there. However, she did not know what fueled this desire, nor did she realize that the plan did not include her. Mr. B. kept this to himself; he did not see this as deceitful nor did he feel guilty.

Mr. B. finished business school and obtained a job in a New York bank. Mrs. B. continued to work although she was eager to become a full-time student and complete her undergraduate education. Soon after moving to New York City, they both expressed satisfaction with their relationship and their life style.

Two months prior to their initial consultation, Mr. B. met a woman he found attractive. He was surprised to find that she encouraged his attentions. Within two or three weeks of that encounter, he told his wife that he had not been sexually attracted to her for the preceding six or more years. This would suggest that he had been attracted to her sexually only for the first six months of their marriage. This surprised Mrs. B. as their sex life had been active and the relationship seemed to her as stable as it had ever been.

Mr. B. presented this to his wife as an unfortunate fact over which he had no control. He did not admit at that point that he wished to separate or be divorced. He simply withdrew from her sexually. Mrs. B. suggested marital therapy hoping that the impasse between them might be resolved. Thus, they came for their initial consultation at New York University Medical Center.

During the initial phases of therapy, Mr. B. was concerned that the goal might be to change the way he felt toward his wife sexually. He stated that to be "cured" of this dissatisfaction was neither desired by him, nor possible. He continued to reiterate his lack of any sexual interest in her. When asked why he had "seemed" to be interested in her sexually for most of the marriage, he stated that he had engaged in sex only out of a sense of duty—this was repeatedly said in a callous, detached and, at times, sadistic manner. During joint sessions he adamantly denied extramarital relationships or interests. However, during an individual session he enthusiastically recounted the story of meeting the other woman.

Our contacts with him were short lived as he continued to make plans to move to the Orient. He seemed no more interested in changing than he was in continuing the relationships with his second wife. Any third marital venture seemed as doomed to failure as the second.

Group Two: The Marriage Phobic

Case 3

C.R. is a 44 year old white divorced male who is presently living alone. He originally sought help in November 1981. His complaints at that time were: (1) that his relationships with women had always deteriorated after a few months of involvement, and (2) he had been fired from his job on one occasion. Since then, although that was many years ago, he was still afraid he might once again be fired. He also noted, "I take myself very seriously—I don't laugh very much." His goals in treatment were to learn how to relate better and to be able to express his anger.

C. was the oldest of two children—he has a sister seven years his junior. His parents were both from families that lived in the same small town in Kansas. After marriage his parents moved several times, eventually settling in an affluent Long Island community when he was 13 years old. He believes the move to Long Island was precipitated by his having been arrested for stealing automobile hub caps in another community.

His parents are deeply troubled individuals. Both are alcoholics—through the years they have had serious marital problems, especially when one or both were drunk. They still live together after almost 50 years of marriage, despite their continuing problems. His mother is a detached, ungiving woman who showed little interest in either of her two children. He requested professional help when in high school so he could have someone with whom to talk. His mother refused, stating, "we are stronger than that." C.'s father was a celebrity in the world of entertainment—C. felt that his father's prominence resulted in problems for him, "I've been under his shadow. Father was at the top of the ladder—that was tough for me." Despite long and repeated absences from home, C.'s father showed more interest in him than did the mother. An example of this disparity was the father's willingness to attend C.'s college graduation while the mother would not. Each parent had occasional affairs. These usually came to light as they handled the affairs in a clumsy, indiscreet manner. The patient has in recent years generously contributed financially to their support.

C.'s father has always been very striving, which may account for his success in a highly competitive field. However, he was as competitive with C. as with all others. Moreover, C.'s successes—and there were many—have rarely been acknowledged by either parent.

C.'s sister has had serious problems—she was in a residential placement for troubled adolescents because of her acting out (fire setting). In addition, she has been in psychotherapy most of her adult life. It was partly the result of her urging that C. sought help.

From an early age C. had serious academic problems—he was diagnosed as dyslexic in the second grade, then had to repeat the eighth grade. He never achieved at a level his superior intellect would indicate was possible. He was twice arrested for theft, first at age 13 and again during his freshman year in college. Being 1500 miles from home in unfamiliar surroundings was a problem for him—he felt lonely, homesick, quite unhappy, and found the adaptation to a new environment most difficult. Until he was in therapy he never connected this episode of stealing with his unhappiness when first away from home. On two separate occasions, despite his loneliness, C. coped with a new and what he perceived to be a hostile environment, with great skill. He decided to become the President of the Student Body in high school and again in college, and was on both occasions successful—both schools were large institutions. In each instance (high school and college) he came to feel that no one knew or respected him. This belief triggered a carefully thought out plan to become better known.

After college he entered the business end of the entertainment world, and was quite successful. However, he lived with the constant dread of being fired. In addition, he had no clear notion as to his career goals.

His relationships with woman have always been quite troubled. What initially would begin as a rewarding and enjoyable experience soon deteriorated into a state of tension and conflict. He dated in high school and college but had no steady girl friends. This pattern continued through his twenties. In the beginning of each new relationship with a woman he would be assertive. He tended to date women who were demanding and dissatisfied. He would try to please the woman and fill her demands. He then would become increasingly compliant. In that setting he stated, "I get quiet." After a few months he would lose all sexual interest in the woman—then he would become impotent.

At the age of 30 he decided it was time he should marry. He soon began to date a girl who had been a classmate in high school and who worked in the same field as he. After a brief courtship they married—this he describes as a "disaster." She was a very impulsive, self-centered woman whose great need to control men was probably the result of her considerable fear of them. She had no intention of having children as this would have interfered with her career plans. They had problems with an intrauterine device that initially seemed to have interfered with their sex life. After a few months his wife expressed growing dissatisfaction with their marriage. She was unhappy with their sex life, but more importantly, found marriage too confining and limiting. One day she precipitously announced her decision to separate and did so 24 hours later. He was devastated by this event—it took him 18 to 24 months to recover emotionally despite the brief duration of their marriage. His wife never remarried in the years following their divorce.

Many months after the divorce, he met the woman with whom he was living at the time he first sought help. After some months of dating, they had decided to live together. He felt less lonely, but he found their bickering troublesome. She complained that he spent more time on his hobbies than on her. She also saw him as stingy and emotionally detached. He found he was constantly trying to please her but was unsuccessful in this effort. Moreover, he found her demanding and unappreciative. Even so, he never became openly angry at her—after a few months their sex life deteriorated. He said, "I have a considerable interest in sex when we are in a dating mode. That interest tends to wane after six months or a year. Then it's every two weeks and when the woman persists. I stop seeing the woman as a lover but rather see her as someone I live with." He also added, "Maybe I have a fatal fickleness."

Eventually she had an affair. When he discovered this, he was again devastated. He soon began an affair with a married co-worker with two children. This was the state of affairs when he first sought help.

Despite his problems with women, C.R. has many good male friends who he saw at regular intervals. Some of these he has known since high school days. Others he met at work. He seems to have a considerable ability to maintain friendships.

He has been seen in weekly psychotherapy for the past 42 months. For many months he was quite defensive of his parents and described them as well adjusted and caring parents. He did not acknowledge their drinking, fighting, selfishness, or inability to show concern or affection. On the other hand, he saw himself as a bad person who poisoned everyone with whom he had dealings. He was very defensive and provided little historical information that would have helped the therapist to understand his situation. In describing himself, he said, "I love the status quo—I'm afraid of any move in any direction." This was certainly true in treatment. Gradually he opened up but progress was slow. As treatment unfolded, it became increasingly clear that C.R. was quite phobic with fears of elevators, small rooms, and any interpersonal situation that he could not control. Any confrontation with others, especially those involving angry feelings, created so much anxiety that he felt an overwhelming need to leave the situation. Hopefully he will make a greater commitment to treatment in the months to come.

C.R. is a very bright 44 year old divorced man whose relationships with women have always been highly conflicted. He is polite, conscientious, and very compliant, especially with women. He is quite anxious in social situations, tends to be shy and retiring despite much charm and a good sense of humor. He prefers to be by himself. Anger is anathema to him. He is quite fearful of new situations and attempts to maintain the status quo. Any risk is something to be avoided—thus he always plays it safe. He has many strengths and has been quite successful in his work despite his constant fear that all he has achieved will be momentarily taken from him. At times, especially with the end of a relationship, he becomes quite depressed—in fact, he holds onto people to avoid the feelings of loss that will result. His relationships with men are much more gratifying than those with women. However, he stated in treatment that he wanted to work toward better relationships with women so that he could meet someone and maintain a long lasting, even permanent, bond with her.

Case 4

P.R. is a 41 year old white man who originally was seen for consultation in February 1974. At that time, he said, "I've always felt not up to snuff. I have a low tolerance for good feelings about myself—I'm more comfortable with bad feelings. In addition, I jump to protect women, not to relate to them." Just prior to the original consultation, he had been in weekly individual therapy on the West Coast. That had been interrupted after one and a half years when he moved to the New York City area as the result of a job change.

During the consultation, the following was noted: "P.R. is the youngest of two with a sister three years his senior. His father died at the age of 42 of rheumatic heart disease when the patient was 4-1/2. The patient has few memories of his father who, prior to his death, owned and managed an art gallery. His mother was from a prominent Texas family. After his father's death, mother and children returned to the home of the patient's maternal grandmother. He grew up in a home dominated by women, especially by his grandmother who he described as a "grand matriarch." He said, "There was no father figure." His older sister was also a powerful force in the home.

He said of his mother, "She had no enemies. I can't respect her—she had no opinions, no viewpoint." His mother died when he was in his mid-twenties. He added as a postscript, "I resent my mother—I see much of her in me." She was a very unhappy person with few interests of her own. She was a large, awkward woman with conspicuous facial scars. These were the result of an auto accident that occurred when she was a young woman.

There were no rules in his grandmother's home—from very early he made important decisions by himself. He was enuretic until he was 10 or 11. This problem prevented him from going to camp and was the cause of great shame. He was, as a boy and adolescent, shy and passive. He decided to go to boarding school at the end of the tenth grade. His high school principal had supported this plan openly, encouraging him to leave home. He was told, "It would be good for you to be away from a female centered house."

He attended an Ivy League college where he made average grades. After graduation he joined the Army and was eventually an officer in the Quartermaster Corp. The structure and rules provided by the Army seemed to fill his needs, thus he was quite happy in service.

After discharge from the Army, he attended a well known school of architecture. He then actively pursued a career in this field, although he never seemed able to make a full commitment to this career. He lived a rather isolated life, first in San Francisco and later in New York City. He had a small group of friends in both cities.

His relationships with women had always been quite troubled. While on the West Coast he dated two women, both of whom made serious suicide attempts while dating him. This act in each instance seemd to stem, at least in part, from their frustrations in relating to him. He seemed unable to make up his mind as to what he wanted of the relationship. He would initially be quite charming and friendly—this would be followed by his suddenly rejecting the woman in a cruel manner. He would then feel guilty and make amends, only to again repeat the cycle. None of his relationships had ever progressed to the point where he and his girl friend were considering marriage. This was the case despite his statement that his goal was to have a wife and family. As soon as he began to view a woman as a potential wife, he would find what he believed was a serious flaw in her.

As a result of the consultation, he was referred to a colleague who worked with him during the next five years. He gained some understanding of his problems with that therapist but made no major changes in the way he was living. He again returned for a consultation in October 1983 when he seemed unable to make a commitment to the woman he had been living with for two years. He then entered treatment and has been seen twice a week since that time.

His prior therapist in New York City had been quite inactive during sessions. He said of him, "He was like my childhood—no rules, no expectations." In the present instance, the therapist

(RMC) concluded that the approach most likely to help him find some direction in life should be challenging and confrontational. Consistent with this approach, his unwillingness to make choices in life and his failure to make commitments were repeatedly interpreted as self-destructive. His intellectualizations were seen as only another means of maintaining the status quo. It was also pointed out to him that he was quite anxious and much of his behavior served the purpose of avoidance—thus he never moved in any direction.

Soon he began to make some choices in life. One of these was to continue to date the girl friend he had been seeing for two years. In October, 1984 he married this young woman. Later he decided to attend graduate school. Both of these decisions, and their subsequent implementation, were times of anxiety with much doubting and postponing. He was tempted to run away. With support from the therapist, he was able to not run and to proceed with the decisions he had made at an earlier time.

He continues in treatment. His marriage is rocky—occasionally he has said he was tempted to leave his wife, expressing doubts of his love for her despite their considerable attachment to one another. He is about to enter graduate school, although he expresses doubts that he will be able to successfully finish school or get a job once graduated.

ANALYSIS OF THE TWO GROUPS

At first blush it would seem that these two groups, The Self Involved Narcissistic Divorce Prone and The Marriage Phobic, would be very different from one another. However, it is our experience that there are some interesting common denominators.

Differences

The particular defensive styles of each group are very different. The Marriage Phobic are very cautious and thus extensively use avoidance as a means of coping with a threatening world. The Self Involved Narcissistic Divorce Prone, on the other hand, are self centered, confident, action oriented, and hard driving. In addition, they are impulsive and reckless—if anything, they are counterphobic. Acting out seems to be their characteristic way of managing conflict and painful emotions.

When it comes to marriage, their defensive styles are immediately apparent.The Divorce Prone, by definition, marry repeatedly, while the Marriage Phobic are the quintessence of caution. Once in a situation, marital or otherwise, the Marriage Phobic stick it out—they find it equally as hard to leave a marriage (or a relationship) as they found it to get into it in the first place. The Marriage Phobic obsess until they have made a decision—then they stick with it. The Divorce Prone quickly decide, act impulsively, but are then ready to change their minds and withdraw from what had originally seemed to be an irrevocable choice.

The Marriage Phobic are usually faithful. C.R. (Case 3) did get involved sexually on one occasion with a co-worker. This was clearly in retaliation for the affair his live-in girl friend had had. The Divorce Prone have affairs while either married or living with someone. They don't seem hobbled by loyalty issues and are all too ready to withdraw from one woman whenever they have "a better offer" from another. Counts and Sacks (1986) stated of this group, "They long for the emotional high of 'being in love' not unlike adolescent infatuations. The idea of being enormously wanted by a new love is something they find irresistible."

The Marriage Phobic, on the other hand, may be drawn to a new love but they are less able to make a move. It's hard to say whether they are constrained by loyalty to their mate or if they are too fearful to act. At times they seem paralyzed by ambivalence and indecisiveness. Although the Marriage Phobic has more guilt feelings than the Divorce Prone, it is our impression they are not necessarily more loyal, just more inhibited and cautious.

The Divorce Prone men seemed to feel remarkably little guilt and had few, if any, regrets. They view their latest divorce as necessary, even inevitable under the circumstances. They expect others to both see it as they do and to be accepting of their explanations. These men get upset when a former mate makes excessive financial demands on them or when she doesn't accept her fate graciously and without protest. They don't seem to feel in any way responsible for the pain experienced by an ex-wife. It is as though they have moved on and thus no longer feel, in any way, responsible for the condition of the ex-mate.

The Marriage Phobic, on the other hand, are more beset by regrets and guilt feelings when a relationship has ended. They often maintain friendly contact with the former mate or girl friend and are a source of support and encouragement to her. The Divorce Prone, in contrast, expect the former mate to remain interested in them and concerned with their welfare. Thus, the Marriage Phobic are supportive of a former mate or girl friend; the Divorce Prone expect to be supported by her.

The Divorce Prone are usually the ones to leave a relationship. This is true of marriage and/or affairs. The Divorce Prone are usually sensitive to any threat of withdrawal by a wife or girl friend. They act first, before she can do so. The Marriage Phobic, on the other hand, find it inordinately hard to leave and often provoke the other person to leave him. C.R. had never initiated the end of a relationship, P.R. had done so rarely. C. R. withdrew into a protective shield of detachment after each abandonment by a woman. When first seen, he was quite depressed. This was apparently a result of his most recent disappointment. He described himself as numb and not interested in beginning any new relationship.

The Divorce Prone were more able to get angry than the Marriage Phobic. While they (the Divorce Prone) were very much in touch with angry feelings, they were not always able to express those feelings openly. Often, when angry, they would withdraw from the old relationship and covertly turn to a new object. However, the women from whom they were withdrawing were not aware they were angry.

The Marriage Phobic, on the other hand, were rarely in touch with their anger and were quite unable to express it directly. In situations usually provocative of anger, they just withdrew into silence and/or depression. Both groups tend to avoid confrontations. Fighting and arguing aren't typical of either of their relationships. B.P.'s third marriage ended in much battling as his wife was very vindictive—he found this experience devastating. She wouldn't allow him to withdraw unless he gave her most of his money and possessions. However, the Divorce Prone were usually quite skillful at avoiding confrontations or "unpleasantness."

The Marriage Phobic would not fight back in an open manner. Despite much abuse, they would just "stand and take it." They seemed to feel that the woman was entitled to this—they would rationalize their mate's or girl friend's behavior and seemed to believe it was their due. They felt deserving of the abuse. They would try, in a very reasoned way, to explain their behavior often to an increasingly irate mate.

The Divorce Prone are more exploitative, even psychopathic, while the Marriage Phobic are more obviously inhibited and fearful.

Similarities

The four men illustrated in these cases utilized intellectualization frequently. It is not clear if this is characteristic of both groups or just of these particular men. Moreover, there were some differences even among these four. It seemed to us that the Marriage Phobic were well rationalized while the Divorce Prone were more ready to give a conventional answer or what they believed the listener expected.

All four of these men saw women (or men friends as well) as engulfing. They dealt with this as noted earlier in this paper. The Divorce Prone make a highly qualified commitment and are quite ready to withdraw, while the Marriage Phobic avoids a feared engulfment by keeping their distance. Both thus avoid engulfment.

While the Divorce Prone seem, in some ways, exploitative and psychopathic, and the Marriage Phobic inhibited and fearful, both groups are equally cautious with women. They see women as threatening and dangerous. While they cope with the fearfulness in different ways, this is an underlying theme. However, if we consider this question from a slightly different angle, these two groups are quite similar. Both are equally fearful of women and do not find them trustworthy. While we define the Marriage Phobic as approaching women in a fearful manner, we might just as appropriately call the Divorce Prone counterphobic in relationship to women. Thus, they may be just as frightened, but approach women in a reckless manner—their gimmick is that rather than committing themselves fully, they make a highly qualified commitment knowing that if things don't pan out they will withdraw. The women don't know this and presume their mate is as committed to the relationship as they. They both need, at all costs, to control women. In this respect both groups are equally successful.

Both groups have considerable problems in making interpersonal decisions and in making a commitment to a relationship. While we initially presumed that these two groups of men would be different in this regard, we came to the conclusion that they were quite similar. The question then is, why is this so? Why do they have a problem in making a commitment? Are all decisions equally difficult for these two groups? Do they see women in a similar light? Are they equally intimidated by women? Do they have similar problems with object constancy?

Perhaps it is in part a mistake to say that the Divorce Prone have difficulty across the board in making decisions. They don't have much difficulty with decisions related to career—in fact, they tend to be innovative and ready to take a lot of initiative. It rather seems that they are free to decide because they are all too ready, in a variety of circumstances, to change their minds. This is true even when it is unusual to change one's mind (with decisions that are normally considered irrevocable).

These two groups do see women in some respects rather differently—the Divorce Prone find it necessary to control women. They do not see women as reliable or trustworthy. However, they tend to be contemptuous of women and are ready to use and exploit them. The Marriage Phobic, on the other hand, are fearful of women, put them on a pedestal, and feel the need to explain their own actions to the women in their lives. The Divorce Prone believe that the woman isn't entitled to an explanation and should not expect one. The woman is expected to accept her fate, whatever that may be. Thus, this group of Divorce Prone tend to be more arrogant.

We find the question of object constancy as pertains to these patients an interesting one. The Marriage Phobic and the Divorce Prone (the Self Involved Narcissist) seem to be on the opposite ends of a spectrum. The Divorce Prone seems ready to change objects at the slightest hint of trouble—the Marriage Phobic stays attached, however much they are abused. They stay in the relationship when to do so seems unwise and self-destructive.

In the earlier study of Divorce Prone (Counts and Sacks, 1986), we described another subcategory of Divorce Prone we called the "Compliant Depressed." They tended, in contrast to the Self Involved Narcissists, to have many fears and inner doubts. Moreover, they respond vigorously to any loss. In these ways, they are similar to the Marriage Phobic. However, the Compliant Depressed are quite different than the Marriage Phobic in one very specific way—they are at times quite impulsive and on occasion have made major life choices without giving the matter much thought. This particular quality leads them into repeated marital failure—the Marriage Phobic, on the other hand, because of a considerable indecisiveness usually avoids this fate. The Compliant Depressed and Marriage Phobic both tend to have a lot of pain.

When it comes to the question of prognosis and treatment outcome, the Marriage Phobic fare better than the Self Involved Narcissistic Divorce Prone. The lack of pain, the self-centeredness, and the fact that the Divorce Prone feel so entitled, interfere with their entering a treatment relationship with any sense of commitment. They are just as lacking in commitment to treatment as they are to a marital relationship. Thus, they are as ready to break off treatment as they are to break off a marriage. This was true of both B.D. and B.P. (Cases 1 and 2). In addition, the Self Involved Narcissistic Divorce Prone feel little pain and see the problem as residing within their mate. Consequent to this, they aren't very ready to enter treatment in the first place.

The Marriage Phobic and the Compliant Depressed Divorce Prone are similar when it comes to treatment. Both are ready to enter and usually have been in psychotherapy on a number of occasions. They also stay in treatment and have a better outcome.

CONCLUSIONS

We have contrasted a subgroup of Divorce Prone men (the Self Involved Narcissist) with men who we have labeled as Marriage Phobic. They are quite different in many aspects. However, they are quite similar in one specific aspect—they are very wary of the opposite sex and feel a great need to be in control of the relationship. The Marriage Phobic maintain control by withholding, the Divorce Prone by making a tentative commitment that they are very ready to withdraw from. Their withdrawal may be triggered by boredom, disappointment, anger, or the availability of a new love object.

REFERENCE

Counts, Robert M. and Sacks, Anita. (1986). Personality Characteristics of Divorce Prone Individuals. *International Journal of Family Therapy*, 1986.

DEFINING THE RANGE OF DYSFUNCTIONAL PATTERNS IN CHILDREN

Children of Divorce: The Question of Clinically Significant Problems

Nancy J. Warren
Eleanor R. Ilgen
Mary E. Van Bourgondien
Judy T. Konanc
Robert S. Grew
Ingrid A. Amara

ABSTRACT. Does divorce typically produce clinically significant problems in children? This paper reports the results of a study of a non-clinical sample of children of divorce using criteria to assess clinically significant levels of problems in school age children. Data gathered 0–4 months after divorce filing (at least 12 months after separation in North Carolina) from 86 families with 112 children aged 7–12 were compared to data from normal reference groups.

Nancy J. Warren, PhD, Eleanor R. Ilgen, MA, MSW, Mary E. Van Bourgondien, PhD, Judy T. Konanc, PhD, and Robert S. Grew, PhD, are on the faculty of the Parenting After Divorce (PAD) Project, Department of Psychiatry, University of North Carolina at Chapel Hill, NC. Ingrid A. Amara, DrPH, is on the faculty of the Department of Biostatistics, University of North Carolina at Chapel Hill, NC.

This research was supported by the National Institute of Mental Health Grant #RO1-34398.

Results showed that divorced and normal school age children were comparable in anxiety, self-esteem, school adjustment and behavior, and family environment. Only parent-reported home behavior problems differed from that for normal comparison groups. Children with clinically significant levels of behavior problems were less likely to have regular visitation and were more likely to have parents in conflict about child rearing. A small group of children with multiple problems appears to be at risk. The results suggest children may adapt to divorce much better than some studies suggest.

Research on families in the midst of divorce and shortly after has produced results which are rich in description. However, they leave unanswered a question central to clinicians: Does divorce typically produce problems in children at levels which are clinically, not just statistically, significant? By not addressing this question, studies of the impact of divorce on children have not served the needs of clinicians as well as they might. This article will attempt to remedy this situation by reporting on the prevalence of clinically significant problems in a sample of children of divorce who participated in the Parenting After Divorce (PAD) Project. The PAD study was undertaken to compare the impact of three different psychoeducational programs (two active and one control) for divorcing families with children aged 7–12. As part of this design objective, the study assessed the prevalence of clinically significant levels of problems in target-age children in participating families just prior to program participation.

Ascertaining the clinical level of problems in children of divorce is important since 40% or more of the children seen in clinics have experienced the separation or divorce of their parents (Kalter & Rembar, 1981). Clinical studies have provided a persuasively detailed picture of problems encountered among children in treatment whose parents were divorced: misbehavior at home and in school, school refusal, depression, delinquency, separation problems, overt aggression and sexual behavior problems (McDermott, 1970; Kalter & Rembar, 1981; Kalter, 1977). Unfortunately, most of the clinical studies typically use retrospective data and poorly defined clinical diagnoses.

Major studies of divorcing families not in treatment (Hetherington, Cox & Cox, 1979; Wallerstein & Kelly, 1974, 1975, 1980; Kelly & Wallerstein, 1976, 1977) also suggest that divorce produces behavioral and affective problems in these children. In addition, studies comparing divorced- and intact-family children have also consistently found small but significant differences between the means of the two groups (Felner, Ginter, Boike & Cowen, 1981; Guidubaldi, Cleminshaw, Perry & Mcloughlin, 1983; Guidubaldi & Perry, 1984; Hetherington, 1979; Hetherington et al., 1979; Jacobson, 1978a, 1978b; Wyman, Cowen, Hightower & Pedro-Carroll, 1985), with children of divorce functioning less well than children from intact families.

Certain methodological constraints have limited the usefulness of information from these studies of non-clinical divorcing families—sampling families who have been referred (Kelly & Berg, 1978; Kurdeck & Seisky, 1980; Wallerstein & Kelly, 1980), using of clinical interviews without support of other measurement tools (Wallerstein & Kelly, 1980), and not taking account of time since the parents physically separated (Guidubaldi et al., 1983; Guidubaldi & Perry, 1984; Jacobson, 1978a,b; Wyman et al., 1985). The most striking omission, however, has been the failure to use clinical norms when discussing problem areas under investigation. Even those studies which have found statistically significant differences between groups of children from divorced and intact families do not report their results with reference to clinical norms. It is therefore unclear whether problems encountered in children of divorce reach clinical levels.

In an effort to shed light on this question, the Parenting After Divorce (PAD) Project is here following the lead of Jacobson and his colleagues (Jacobson, Follette & Revenstorf, 1984; Jacobson, Follette, Revenstorf, Baucom, Hahlweg & Margolin, 1984; Jacobson & Follette, 1985), who are conducting outcome research focusing on clinically significant change in family and marital therapy. Criteria for describing clinical problem levels (Jacobson et al., 1984) guided the development of a strategy for determining clinical levels of problems in the study sample of 112 school-age children of divorce. Established clinical cutoff scores, or means and standard deviations established for each test, were used to indicate functioning in the normal or clinical problem range. The proportion of children functioning in the clinical problem range was then calculated for each standardized test of functioning used (see Method section below). This paper will describe the results of this effort, which was designed to determine the extent of clinically significant problems in these children at the time their parents filed for divorce.

METHOD

Sample

The eligible study population was defined as all families having at least one child aged 7–12 and filing for divorce in a four-county area in central North Carolina between September 1980 and May 1983. Under North Carolina law, couples must have been separated at least 12 months in order to file for divorce. Thus all eligible families, who were identified from court records, were contacted at least a year beyond the point of physical separation. Though there is no stipulated maximum length of separation before filing for divorce, families in which the parents had been separated for more than four years were excluded from the study.

The residential (custodial) parent and children were contacted within four months of the divorce filing and invited to participate in three three-hour testing sessions (over a period of one year) and a six-week educational program. Although subjects were not paid, the programs were offered free of charge. Informed consent was obtained from the parent and the children before testing began.

Table 1 shows the results of sample recruitment. The acceptance rate achieved is similar to that obtained in other studies of divorcing families (Kalter, personal communication, 1984). Also, because the

TABLE 1

SAMPLE RECRUITMENT

	n	%
No contact possible	587	36.2%
Letter only	541	33.4%
Letter and telephone contact	492	30.4%
	1620	100.0%
Response of those contacted (n=492)		
Decline participation	272	55.3%
Ineligible (child out of area, in treatment, wrong age)	77	15.6%
Agreed, did not follow through	57	11.6%
Agreed, pretested	86	17.5%
	492	100.0%

focus of the study was on the impact of divorce on children whose families could benefit from educational parenting programs without therapeutic support for the child, families were excluded if *all* target age children were currently in treatment. It should be noted that, out of the total 492 eligible families reached by phone, only 26 (5.3%) were excluded for this reason.

The study sample consists of 86 families with 112 children between the ages of 7–12: 51 children aged 7–9 and 61 children aged 10–12. Fifteen children (13.4%) had received some counseling prior to participating in the study. An additional four (3.6%) were currently in treatment but had target-age siblings who were not. Additional characteristics of the sample are presented in Table 2.

Potential sources of bias in the sample were assessed by comparing the sample (n = 86) with the eligible nonparticipating families (n = 1534). The results of this comparison are presented in Table 2, which indicates that the findings of the PAD sample are limited in their applicability largely to white families and to those black families who are somewhat more financially stable and less mobile than those not studied. Since national figures are not available on divorcing families with children in the age range targeted by this study, it is impossible to know how the study sample differs from divorced/divorcing families with children in the 7–12 age group living elsewhere.[1]

Measures

The adjustment of children in participating families was evaluated by several different measures. Table 3 presents a list of the measures, subscales used, reference populations, and cutoff scores. In light of the emphasis in this paper on clinically significant problems, particular attention will be paid to a description of the normative population and cut-off scores for each measure.

Measures completed by the children themselves include the Self Observation Scales (SOS; Stenner and Katzenmeyer, 1979). The scale was tested extensively with a sample of 30,000 normal school children in grades K–6, with excellent reliability and validity reported.[2] Also completed by the children, the Children's Manifest Anxiety Scale-Revised (Reynolds & Richmond, 1978) is a 37-item True-False test. Although this measure was tested on a much smaller number of normal school children (n = 329) than the SOS, psychometric studies on the test are adequate. The reliability

TABLE 2

Characteristics of Participating (PAD) and Nonparticipating Families

	PAD (n=86)	Nonparticipating (n=1534)	p
Race	15.48%	25.53%	.038
# of children/family	2	2	ns
Average age of minor children	9.81 years	9.54 years	ns
Marriage to physical separation	11.48 years	10.48 years	.018
Physical separation to filing	14.39 months	17.21 months	.003
Filing to divorce	1.67 months	1.61 months	ns
Amount of child support/child/month	$173	$141	.024
Families with a premarital conception	11.11%	19.60%	.082
Families with a premarital birth	11.11%	13.24%	ns
Families with joint legal custody	20.31%	7.27%	.001
Families in which father filed for divorce	47.56%	43.07%	ns
Plaintiff represented by lawyer	90.77%	87.67%	ns
Primary parent:		not available	
Mother	92.0%		
Father	8.0%		
Socioeconomic status:		not available	
Class I	1.2%		
Class II	24.8%		
Class III	53.0%		
Class IV	21.0%		
Class V	0.0%		

coefficient is reported as .85 and studies show a correlation with other measures of trait anxiety (Reynolds, 1980).

The Moos Family Environment Scale (Moos, Insel & Humphrey, 1974, 1981) was given to all children age 10 and over. The scale has been tested with normal families (n = 1125) and several different groups of distressed families (n = 458).[3] Means and standard deviations for normal families were used in the analysis. Test-retest reliability coefficients range from a low of .68 to .86. The fact that clinic and nonclinic families score differently on the measure has been used to support its construct validity.

Residential parents completed the Eyberg Child Behavior Inventory (ECBI) for each of their children (Eyberg & Ross, 1978; Robinson, Eyberg & Ross, 1980; Eyberg & Robinson, 1983). The ECBI is a 36-item scale which assesses the number and frequency (intensity) of conduct problem behaviors in children 2–16. It was first developed in Oregon with a relatively low SES non-clinical pediatric sample (n = 700) that was stratified by age and sex. Test-retest reliability coefficients have been reported as .86 for the intensity scale and .88 for the problem scale. The measure has been shown to discriminate between normal and conduct problem chil-

TABLE 3

Measures

Measure	Reference Population	Subscales Used	Cutoff Score
Self Observation Scales (SOS) (Stenner and Katzenmeyer, 1979)	1a,2,3,4,5,6	Self-acceptance, self confidence and security, social maturity and school affiliation	1SD = T Score ≤ 40 2SD = T Score < 30
Eyberg Child Behavior Inventory (ECBI) (Robinson, Eyberg, & Ross, 1980)	1a,1b,3,4	Frequency of problem behaviors (ECBI-I) and # of different problem areas (ECBI-P)	Intensity > 127 No. of Problems ≥ 11
Children's Manifest Anxiety Scale-Revised (CMAS-R) (Reynolds **& Richmond,** 1978)	1a,3,4	Anxiety (CMAS-A) & defensiveness (lie) (CMAS-L)	Lie Scale: (7-9) l ≥ 7; (10-12) l > 5 Anxiety Scale: (7-9) l ≥ 22; (10-12) l ≥ 1
Family Environment Scale (FES) (Moos, Insel, and Humphrey,1974)	1a,1b,4,6	Cohesion, conflict, expressiveness, organization, control, & incongruency	Cohe: 1=T Score≤40; 2=T Score≤30 Expr: 1=T Score≤40; 2=T Score<30 Conf: 1=T Score≥60; 2=T Score>70 Org: 1=T Score<40; 2=T Score<30 Con: 1=T Score≥60; 2=T Score>70
National Health Survey School Questionnaire (National Center for Health Statistics, 1972)	1a,2,3,4,5,6	Academic performance, behavior problems in school, and school adjustment	
Family Interaction Scale (FIRS) (Warren & Van Bourgondien,1983)		Global adjustment; family atmosphere; parent consistency, control involvement, and affect; child role, maturity, activity, and affect	

1a = non-clinical sample
1b = clinical sample
2 = sample obtained from vast geographical area
3 = sample stratified by age
4 = sample stratified by sex
5 = sample stratified by SES
6 = sample stratified by race

dren, and the authors provide cutoff scores for use in clinical settings (Eyberg & Ross, 1978).

For a more objective view of the children, each child's teacher was asked to complete a school questionnaire originally used in the National Health Survey (1972). This scale has been used with a national probability sample of 7,119 children, and norms for children aged 6–11 are available. Return rate for the school questionnaire in the present study was 77%.

Family play interactions were videotaped and rated by means of a system developed for the present study, the Family Interaction Rating System (FIRS). Families were videotaped for 30 minutes while they played with Childcraft blocks and Chinese checkers. Ratings using the FIRS had excellent rater agreement, and high correlations with other measures of child adjustment (Warren & Van Bourgondien, unpublished data) but no norm group comparisons with nondivorced family interactions are yet available.[3] The FIRS findings will be reported only to augment findings about the children derived from the other measures.

Finally, to assess the association between child functioning and post-divorce family variables, information was gathered from each parent in an extensive semi-structured interview about family background and divorce-related life events, including details about custody, visitation, and the non-residential parent's involvement in raising the children.

Data Analysis Methods

Each child's score on each measure of child functioning used in the PAD study was classified as either in the normal or in the clinical problem range for that measure. With the exception of the School Questionnaire, scores in the *normal range* were defined as (1) those within one standard deviation of the mean developed for that measure from information provided about the various reference populations used to norm the measure (SOS, FES, and CMAS-R), or (2) those below the clinical cutoff score reported for the measure (ECBI). Scores in the *clinical problem range* were defined as (1) those at least one standard deviation from the mean in the deviant direction or (2) at or above the clinical cutoff score. Where possible within the clinical problem range, scores 1SD from the mean were distinguished from those 2SD from the mean. For the School

Questionnaire, the definition of normal and abnormal behavior provided in the answer checklist for each item was used.

The percentage of children with scores in the normal or clinical problem range was then computed for each measure. A z statistic was then used to compare the percentage of PAD children with problematic scores on a given measure to a standard percentage expected to have problems on that measure. With the exception of the School Questionnaire (National Health Survey), the percentage of reference population children with problems was not indicated. However, under the assumption of the normal distribution, the percentage of test scores 1SD in the deviant direction from the mean is 16%. Thus, 16% was used as the standard percentage for these measures. The National Health Survey provided information about the percentage of children having problems item by item. These percentages were used as the standard percentages in the analysis of the School Questionnaire data. The analysis was designed to indicate significant differences between PAD children and the reference populations only with regard to the percentage of children with clinically significant problems. It did not attempt to detect differences between the sample children and reference populations as to the overall distribution of the children's test scores.

Spearman rank correlation probabilities were used to assess associations between child functioning and family background variables. Variables investigated included such things as SES, involvement of the non-custodial parent in the life of the child, degree of parental agreement about child rearing, amount of disagreement about custody, visitation and other divorce-related issues, frequency of visitation, contact with grandparents, and number and ages of siblings.

RESULTS

Table 4 shows the proportions of children age 7–9 functioning in the normal and clinical problem range for each of the measures, while Table 5 presents these findings for children age 10–12. Both age groups of children show no more anxiety than other school children their age (CMAS-A), nor are they more defensive than expected (CMAS-L). Further, the children show no more problems with self-esteem than a national sample of normal school children on three of the four Self Observation Scales. On the intensity scale

TABLE 4

Functioning of PAD sample children
compared to established norm groups

Children Age 7–9 (n=47)

	Normal	1SD	2SD	Z score	p *
CMAS-R Anxiety	88%	12%	0%	-0.79	ns
CMAS-R Lie	74%	26%	0%	1.46	ns
ECBI Intensity	71%	29%	---	1.96	<.05
ECBI Problems	52%	48%	--	4.28	<.01
SOS Self Acceptance	91%	3%	6%	-1.65	ns
SOS Social Maturity	97%	3%	---	-5.17	ns
SOS School Affiliation	79%	15%	6%	0.83	ns
SOS Self Security	94%	3%	3%	-2.86	ns

* Z=1.65, p<.10
Z=1.96, p<.05
Z=2.58, p<.01

of the Eyberg Child Behavior Inventory (ECBI-I), parent-reported problematic behavior in the 10–12 year olds occurred at a rate comparable to that for normal children (Eyberg and Ross, 1978), with 78% of the 10–12 year old children scoring in the acceptable range.

In the area of school functioning (Table 6), the 7–12 year olds in the PAD sample demonstrate the same pattern of problem behaviors as the group of normal children included in the National Health Survey. The percentage with problem behaviors does not differ significantly between the two samples.

In the area of family functioning, a similar functioning status is found for the children. On the Family Environment Scale (FES), the percentage of PAD children age 10–12 who rate their families as non-distressed on conflict, family cohesion, control and family organization is not statistically different from the percentage expected, although three of the four percentages exceed 16% (see Table 4). Children aged 7–9 did not complete the FES.

Supporting information from ratings of family interaction on the videotapes is as follows: Seventeen percent of the families were rated as functioning less than adequately on overall family adjustment by independent raters (Figure 1), while child affect was rated as happy/appropriate to the play situation rather than tense, sad or angry. Children were also rated as generally age-appropriate in their activity level, maturity, responsibility-taking, and cooperation.

Children's scores on only three measures are not statistically within clinically normal limits. Forty-eight percent of the children 7–9 and 44% of the children 10–12 have a clinically significant number (i.e., > = 11) of problem behaviors at home as rated by

TABLE 5

Functioning of PAD sample children

Compared to established norm groups

Children aged 10–12 (n=54)

	Normal	1SD	2SD	Z Score	p *
CMAS-R Anxiety	88%	12%	0%	-0.88	ns
CMAS-R Lie	80%	20%	0%	0.71	ns
ECBI Intensity	78%	22%	---	1.05	ns
ECBI Problems	56%	44%	---	4.03	<.01
SOS Self Acceptance	80%	15%	5%	0.73	ns
SOS Social Maturity	85%	6%	9%	-0.19	ns
SOS School Affiliation	73%	17%	10%	1.82	<.10
SOS Self Security	90%	5%	5%	-1.47	ns
FES Cohesion	88%	5%	7%	-0.90	ns
FES Expressiveness	36%	49%	15%	7.35	<.01
FES Conflict	83%	15%	2%	0.20	ns
FES Organization	78%	17%	5%	1.06	ns
FES Control	73%	24%	3%	1.82	<.10
FES Parent: Child Incongruency	63%	27%	10%	3.14	<.01

* Z=1.65, p<.10
Z=1.96, p<.05
Z=2.58, p<.01

Table 6

School Functioning of PAD children

Compared to the National Health Survey (1972) Sample

7-9 Year Olds

	PAD%	NHS%	Z
Ajustment Problems	21.21%	16.5%	.6615
Lack of Attentiveness	22.86%	21.37%	.2099
Excessive Motor Activity	15.15%	8.0%	1.1460
Frequently Accused of Fighting	3.85%	6.77%	-.8440
Excessive Rough Play	3.85%	5.27%	-.415
Aggression Makes Discipline Necessary	6.63%	6.70%	-.015

10-12 Year Olds

	PAD%	NHS%	Z
Adjustment Problems	25.53%	18.1%	1.168
Lack of Attentiveness	32.60%	22.60%	1.447
Excessive Motor Activity	11.46%	8.15%	.704
Frequently Accused of Fighting	3.34%	6.35%	-1.123
Excessive Rough Play	5.00%	4.95%	.015
Aggression Makes Discipline Necessary	11.67%	7.65%	.839

No comparisons were significant at the $p < .05$ level

parents on the ECBI-P number of problems scale (Eyberg & Ross, 1978). Further, the younger children are more likely than expected to misbehave more frequently (ECBI-I). In addition, slightly more of the older children than expected also scored in the problem range on the SOS school affiliation scale (27% of those 10–12, $p < .10$). The 10–12 year olds also report significantly less expressiveness and significantly more disagreement with their parents' perceptions

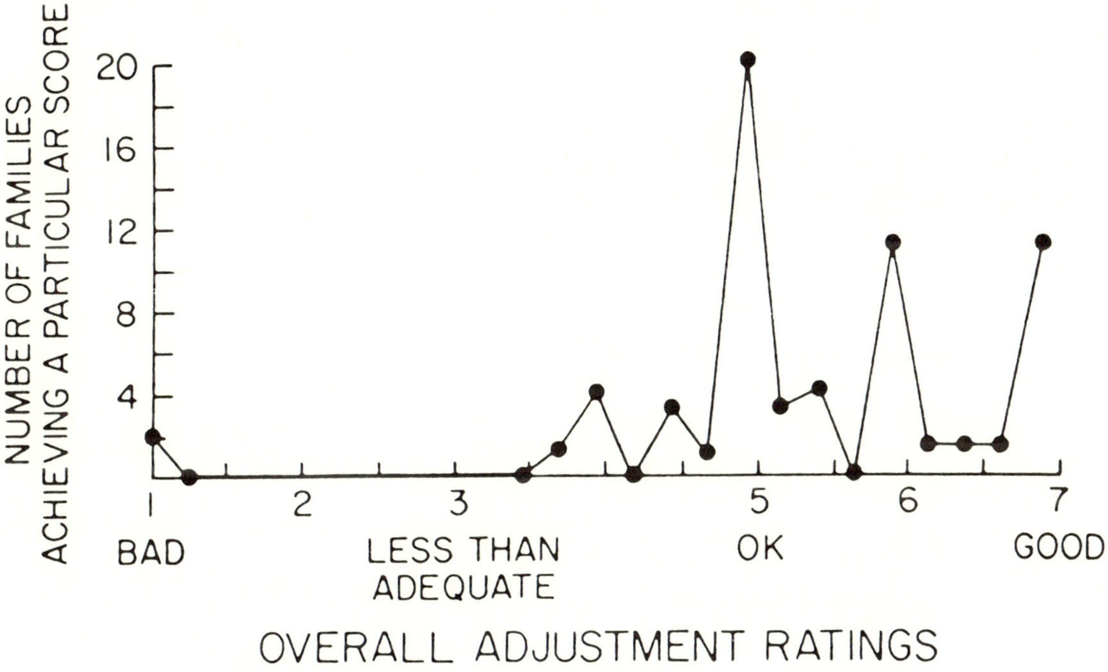

FIGURE 1. Overall Family Adjustment Ratings Family Videotape Observation

of their families on the FES than the reference group families. However, Moos (1981, Appendix E, p. 38) notes that adolescents tend to score below their parents on ratings of expressiveness, even in non-distressed families.

Correlations between problems and divorce-related family life variables were calculated to clarify the background differences between children without clinical problems on the ECBI and those with clinical problems. A closer look at Table 7 reveals that, for children 7–9, statistically significant correlations were found between ECBI-I scores and post-separation family life. Children aged 7–9 with clinically problematic ECBI-I scores live in families in which there are more older children, particularly more boys 10–12 years old. In addition, these children have more contact with their non-custodial parent's family before the separation than after it, and more contact with their custodial parent's family since the separation.

For children aged 10–12, significant correlations were found between ECBI-P scores and family life. Children aged 10–12 with 11 or more problem behaviors are more likely than children with fewer problems to have their non-custodial parent less involved in their upbringing, their parents less in agreement about issues regarding the children, and the parent with whom they live less satisfied with the coparenting relationship. These children also see their second parent less frequently than children with fewer problem behaviors. High ECBI-I scores were also associated with less agreement between parents for the 10–12 year olds.

DISCUSSION

Results of the PAD study show that, although problems are seen in parent ratings of home behaviors and family incongruency, PAD study children are not functioning outside of normal limits on self esteem, anxiety, defensiveness and school adjustment and behavior. This statistically-based finding should be understood within the context of the fact that, on several of the measures, the percentage of PAD children with problems did exceed the expected rate slightly (see Tables 4–6). In the balance, however, these results suggest that, although children of divorce are at risk, it cannot be assumed that all children of divorce are in need of clinical intervention. Further, the normal functioning of some children of divorce cannot

Table 7

Correlations Between Eyberg Problems and Family Life Variables

7-9 year olds

ECBI-I Scale	Family Variable	r	p
	Amount of contact with non-custodial parents family now as compared with before separation	.372	<.05
	Amount of contact with custodial parent's family since separation	.339	<.05
	Number of children in family	.228	<.05
	Number of boys in family	.228	<.05

10-12 year olds

ECBI-P Scale	Family Variable	r	p
	Amount of agreement between parents	-.574	<.001
	Custodial parent's satisfaction with the coparenting arrangement	-.385	<.01
	Frequency of visitation	-.337	<.05
	Amount of non-custodial parent's involvement in parenting since the separation	-.303	<.05

be dismissed merely as evidence of denial or other troubling defenses. On both the objective measures and clinical ratings of family interactions, the majority of children show consistent evidence of resiliency and adaptation.

How can these findings of unexpectedly low rates of clinical problems be reconciled with those of other studies? First, as noted earlier, most other studies have not attempted to assess clinically significant levels of problems when studying the adjustment of children of divorce. The differences reported between divorced and intact family children thus may not reflect *clinically* significant differences in functioning for most children.

Second, time since separation is an important factor. Families in the present study had been separated an average of 14.4 months when they were evaluated. Studies which assess children immediately after parental separation (Wallerstein & Kelly, 1975; Kelly & Wallerstein, 1976) or which do not analyze their data with reference to time since separation (Guidubaldi et al., 1984), tend to report more problems in the children than are reported here. By contrast, studies which followed children over time (Hetherington, 1979; Wallerstein & Kelly, 1980; Wallerstein, 1984) or assess children later in the divorce process (Hess & Camara, 1979) find lower rates of problems by two or three years following the parents' separation.

A Subgroup at Risk

Another important finding of the PAD study, however, is that there is clearly a subgroup of children who are functioning poorly more than a year after separation. Children who have problems in home behaviors (ECBI-P) constitute a mixed group—approximately half (54%) of those with clinically significant ECBI-P scores have no other problems, while the other half (46%) were found to have problems in two or more other areas. Despite being at risk, few of these children had been in treatment.

Since children from divorced homes are typically referred to treatment long after the parental separation—as much as 4–5 years later (Kalter & Rembar, 1981)—it is extremely important to study early risk factors. The variables associated with children's behavioral and school problems an average of 14 months after separation found in this study include disagreement between parents about child rearing, disagreement about the custody arrangement, less involvement in parenting by the non-resident parent, less visitation, and interestingly enough, increased contact with the residential parent's extended family. Like other studies (Hetherington, 1979; Hess & Camara, 1979), these data suggest that children's increased distress may result, not from divorce per se, but from unsatisfactory post-divorce arrangements.

Limitations of the Study

Some of this study's limitations affect the interpretation of its major finding that an unexpectedly small percentage of children in the study sample have clinical problems. First, the children come from families who are predominantly white and generally more financially secure than eligible families who did not participate (see Table 2). In this regard, the study is like most of the divorce studies reported in the literature, including the major ones (Hetherington, 1979; Wallerstein & Kelly, 1980). Since this kind of sample may result in an under-estimation of the proportion of children with clinical problem levels (Brandwein, Brown, & Fox, 1974), the rates of clinical problems reported here may need to be adjusted upwards.

Second, the study's emphasis on preventive education produced a study sample in which only a small percentage (3.6%) of the children were in clinical treatment at the time they were assessed. While there is no guarantee that children from divorcing families enter treatment because they have clinical levels of problems, it seems reasonable to suggest that a sample with a larger number of children in treatment might result in a higher rate of clinical problems. For this reason, too, the rates reported here may need to be adjusted upwards.

Finally, the study was conducted in a state where divorcing parties cannot file for divorce until they have been physically separated for at least one year. As a result, this article reports on problems in children who were assessed an average of 14 months after their parents physically separated. It does not provide information about the children's functioning during the immediate post-separation period, when the rate of clinical problems may well be higher.

Areas for Future Research

In light of these limitations, this article should be seen as a first attempt to address the issue of obtaining clinically meaningful results in research on the effects of divorce on children. By overcoming the limitations, future research can clarify and correct the picture of clinical problem rates presented here.

Adequate representation of black and lower SES families will permit the development of broadly applicable generalizations about the level of clinical problems in children of divorce. So, too, will the inclusion of a representative number of children of divorce in treatment. Since time since separation is an important factor in a child's adjustment, research on clinical problem levels also needs to be conducted in states with divorce laws not requiring a one-year physical separation before filing, thus permitting the identification of a naturalistic sample of divorcing families close to the time of the parents' physical separation. The use of a group of matched controls from intact families will allow researchers and clinicians to see more clearly how children of divorce from otherwise similar children as far as the prevalence of clinical problems is concerned.

The major need here, however, is for the development of a working consensus about the level of problems which should be considered clinically significant (Jacobson et al., 1985). Jacobson recommends a criterion of 2SD beyond the mean. While this permits a clear differentiation of clinical from non-clinical populations, the criterion is set too high for those whose goals are preventive. In the present study, for example, the more conservative norm of 1SD was used because it permitted identification of children who were not flagrantly poor functioning nor yet in treatment but were nevertheless thought to be sufficiently symptomatic as to warrant clinical concern. Until a consensus is reached, those with other goals might use different criteria.

Regardless of the criteria used, however, the long-term clinical effects of divorce on children cannot be understood until the criteria have been applied to longitudinal data within a complex network of situational information about divorcing and post-divorce families. The results reported here show a nonclinical community sample of school-age children of divorce generally with no more clinical problems than other populations of children at approximately 14 months after their parents' physical separation. A three-to-five year follow-up assessment of study families, now underway, is exploring whether these initial results hold up over time. Results of this followup study which will be reported in future papers, should help clarify further some of the issues raised here.

NOTES

1. National figures, which are derived by the National Center for Health Statistics from information reported by 31 states, make no distinction between childless divorcing couples and those who have any minor children. Thus, there exists no national statistical profile of divorcing families with minor children of any age.

2. Test-retest reliability for the Primary scale ranged from .79 to .91 with .86 as the median. The Intermediate scale also had excellent reliability with the range being .73 to .89 and the median being .85. The authors support the construct and intrinsic validity of the scales by demonstrating the replicability invariance and constancy of the correlation coefficients across a wide range of criterion groups. Support for the extrinsic validity of the scale comes from a variety of sources. Stenner and Katzenmeyer (1979) found that each of the scales was positively related to rated reading achievement beyond the .001 level. Positive correlations between self-concept, emotional adjustment, and academic achievement have been shown in other studies (Williams and Cole, 1968).

3. The interrater reliability on 9 of the 11 scales ranged from 70% to 86%. Two scales had relatively poor reliability: Parent Consistency, 53% and Child Affect, 60%. Raters were ignorant of the treatment condition of families in the study.

REFERENCES

Brandwein, R. A., Brown, C. A., & Fox, E. M. (1974). Women and children lost: The social situation of divorced mothers and their families. *Journal of Marriage and the Family, 36*, 498–514.

Bloom, B. L. & Hodges, W. F. (1978). *The Background Information Questionnaire* (BIQ). Unpublished manuscript, University of Colorado, Boulder.

Eyberg, S. M., & Robinson, E. A. (1983). Conduct problem behavior: Standardization of a behavior rating scale with adolescents. *Journal of Clinical Child Psychology, 12*, 347–354.

Eyberg, S. M., & Ross, A. W. (1978). Assessment of child behavior problems. The validation of new inventory. *Journal of Clinical Child Psychology, 7*, 113–116.

Felner, R. D., Ginter, M. A., Boike, M. F., & Cowen, E. L. (1981). Parental death or divorce and the school adjustment of young children. *American Journal of Community Psychology, 9*, 181–191.

Guidubaldi, J., Cleminshaw, H. K., Perry, J. D., & Mcloughlin. (1983). The impact of parental divorce on children: Report of a nationwide NASP study. *School Psychology Review, 12*, 300–323.

Guidubaldi, J., & Perry, J. D. (1984). Divorce, socioeconomic status and children's cognitive-social competence at school entry. *American Journal of Orthopsychiatry, 54*, 459–468.

Hess, R., & Camara, K. (1979). Post-divorce family relationships as mediating factors in the consequences of divorce for children. *Journal of Social Issues, 35*, 79–96.

Hetherington, E. (1979). Divorce: a child's perspective. *American Psychologist, 34*, 851–858.

Hetherington, E., Cox, M., & Cox, R. (1979). Play and social interaction in children following divorce. *Journal of Social Issues, 35*, 26–49.

Jacobson, D. S. (1978). The impact of marital separation/divorce on children: I. Parent-child separation and child adjustment. *Journal of Divorce, 1*, 341–359.

Jacobson, D. S. (1978). The impact of marital separation/divorce on children: II. Interparent hostility and child adjustment. *Journal of Divorce, 2*, 3–20.

Jacobson, N. S., & Follette, W. C. (1985). Clinical significance of improvement resulting from two behavioral marital components. *Behavior Therapy, 16*, 249–262.

Jacobson, N. S., Follette, W. C., & Revenstorf, D. (1984). Psychotherapy outcome research: Methods for reporting variability and evaluating clinical significance. *Behavior Therapy, 15*, 336–352.

Jacobson, N. S., Follette, W. C., Revenstorf, D., Baucom, D. H., Hahlweg, K., & Margolin, G. (1984). Variability in outcome and clinical significance of behavioral

marital therapy: A reanalysis of outcome data. *Journal of Consulting and Clinical Psychology, 51*, 497–504.
Kalter, N. (1977). Children of divorce in an outpatient psychiatric population. *American Journal of Orthopsychiatry, 47*, 40–51.
Kalter, N., & Rembar, J. (1981). The significance of child's age at the time of parental divorce. *American Journal of Orthopsychiatry, 51*, 85–100.
Kelly, J. B. & Wallerstein, J. S. (1976). The effects of parental divorce: experiences of the child in early latency. *American Journal of Orthopsychiatry, 46*, 20–32.
Kelly, J. B., & Wallerstein, J. S. (1977). Part-time child: visiting after divorce. *Journal of Clinical Child Psychology, 6*, 51–54.
Kelly, R. & Berg, S. (1978). Measuring children's reactions to divorce. *Journal of Clinical Psychology, 34*, 215–221.
Kurdeck. L. A., & Seisky, A. E. (1980). Effects of divorce on children: the relationship between parent and child perspective. *Journal of Divorce, 4*, 85–99.
Landis, J. R., & Koch, G. G. (1979). The analysis of categorical data in longitudinal studies of behavior development. In J. R. Nesselroade and P. B. Baltes (Eds.), *Longitudinal Research in the Study of Behavior and Development* (pp. 233–261). New York: Academic Press.
McDermott, J. F. (1970). Divorce and its psychiatric sequellae in children. *Archives of General Psychiatry, 23*, 421–427.
Moos, R. H., Insel, D. M., & Humphrey, B. (1974). *Preliminary Manual for Family Environment Scale, Work Environment Scale, Group Environment Scale*. Palo Alto, CA: Consulting Psychologists Press.
Moos, R. H., Insel, D. M., & Humphrey, B. (1981). *Family Environment Scale*. Palo Alto, CA: Consulting Psychologists Press.
Reynolds, C. R. (1980). Concurrent validity of what I think and feel: The revised Children's Manifest Anxiety Scale. *Journal of Consulting and Clinical Psychology, 48*, 774–775.
Reynolds, C. R., & Richmond, B. O. (1978). What I think and feel: A revised measure of children's manifest anxiety. *Journal of Abnormal Child Psychology, 6*, 271–280.
Robinson, E. A., Eyberg, S. M., & Ross, A. W. (1980). The standardization of an inventory of child conduct problem behaviors. *Journal of Clinical Child Psychology*, Spring, 22–29.
Stenner, A. J. & Katzenmeyer, W. G. (1979). *Self Observation Scales: Technical Manual and users guide*. Durham, NC: NTS Research Corporation.
Wallerstein, J. S., & Kelly, J. B. (1974). The effects of parental divorce: the adolescent experience. In E. Anthony and C. Kopernik (Eds.), *The Child and His Family: Children at Psychiatric Risk* (Vol. 3).
Wallerstein, J. S., & Kelly, J. B. (1975). The effects of parental divorce: experiences of the pre-school child. *Journal of the American Academy of Child Psychiatry, 14*, 600–616.
Wallerstein, J. S. & Kelly, J. B. (1980). *Surviving the Breakup: How Children and Parents Cope with Divorce*. New York: Basic Books.
Warren, N. J. & Van Bourgondien, M. E. (1983). *Family Interaction Rating System (FIRS): Coding manual and clinical rating form*. Unpublished manuscript, University of North Carolina, School of Medicine, Chapel Hill.
Williams, R. L. & Cole, S. (1968). Self-concept and school adjustment. *Personnel and Guidance Journal, 78*, 478–481.
Wyman, P. A., Cowen, E. L., Hightower, A. D., & Pedro-Carroll, J. L. (1985). Perceived competence, self-esteem, and anxiety in latency aged children of divorce. *Journal of Clinical Child Psychology, 14*, 20–26.

Who Are the "Normal" Children of Divorce? On the Need to Specify Population

Marla B. Isaacs
George Leon
Ann Marie Donohue

ABSTRACT. There is a growing body of literature on the effects of marital dissolution on the adjustment of children. A weakness of many empirical studies, however, is the tendency to gather data on families who have requested counseling and to assume that results from such a sample may be generalized to all separating families. This can lead researchers and clinicians to ignore important differences that may exist between separating families who have requested counseling and those who have not.

The present study addresses this problem by examining a sample of approximately one hundred divorcing families, half of whom have requested counseling and half have not. Standardized tests of adjustment were used to assess the children's adjustment and the results were compared to scores of a standardized "normal" and "clinical" sample. The results indicate that the sample of children undergoing parental separation does not conform to a simple normal-clinical dichotomy. It was also found that significant differences in adjustment exist between the children of those families who had requested counseling and those who had not.

The dissolution of parents' marriage has been ranked as one of the major sources of stress for children (Holmes and Rahe, 1967) and rising divorce rates have prompted a growing body of research to investigate the impact of parental separation on children's mental health (Wallerstein and Kelly, 1980; Hetherington, 1972; Hether-

Marla B. Isaacs, PhD, George Leon, PhD, and Ann Marie Donohue, PhD, are on the staff of the Families of Divorce Project, Philadelphia Child Guidance Clinic, Two Children's Center, 34 Street and Civic Center Boulevard, Philadelphia, PA 19104.

ington et al., 1978; Goetting, 1981; Isaacs, 1985). However, current divorce research has not addressed the possibility of differences in adjustment between families that have requested counseling or therapy following separation and those that have not. Since clinic-referral in general is an important predictor of persistent problems for children (Achenbach and Edelbrock, 1981), failure to take counseling into account in divorce research may result in findings about child adjustment that are misleading. The purpose of the present study is to explore this issue by comparing the adjustment of children from families who have requested counseling to those who have not.

Findings in the divorce literature to date point to the first post-separation year as one in which a majority of children are prone to show emotional or behavioral difficulties of some kind, although there is less agreement across studies as to the probability of longer term effects (Wallerstein and Kelly, 1980; Hetherington et al., 1978; Young and Parish, 1979; McDermott, 1971; Kulka and Weingarten, 1979; Hodges et al., 1979). In most of these investigations the presence of emotional difficulties has been determined by differential comparisons across groups of children from various family types, such as happy intact families, conflictual intact families, divorced or widowed single parents and so on, or else by within-group variations in the nature and severity of difficulties among children of divorced parents (Hetherington et al., 1978; Young and Parish, 1979; McDermott, 1971; Kulka and Weingarten, 1979; Hodges et al., 1979.) Several studies have revealed differences in adjustment between boys and girls and among children of different ages (Hetherington et al., 1978, McDermott, 1968; Wallerstein and Kelly, 1980; Santrock and Warshak, 1979). These procedures, although quite appropriate to the purposes of divorce research, leave unclear the extent to which problems thus identified mirror those found in what the psychopathology literature would describe as a "clinical" group. In other words, these approaches may make it possible to say whether children of divorce display problem behaviors sufficient to distinguish them from a randomly-chosen sample of normal children, but do not permit conclusions as to their similarity to a clinically-disturbed population. It is conceivable, for example, that the response of many children to parental separation may be characterized by a pattern of marked, but transient, symptomatic behaviors that would extend the conventional clinical-normal dichotomy to include a third group, such as "children under stress." By including both "clinical" and "normal" group comparisons, divorce researchers may provide empirical support, and much-needed refinement, for this important grouping.

The selection of appropriate samples for the study of children's post-separation adjustment might also be informed by current practice in the diagnostic literature. Achenbach and Edelbrock (1981) have noted that the criterion of clinic-referral is one of the best available indicators of persisting childhood problems. Yet, in the divorce research, there has been a tendency to treat as equally representative of all children of divorcing parents, those whose families are in divorce-related counseling or support groups, and those who are not. This practice implies that children undergoing the stress of divorce are expected to be more similar to one another than to their counterparts in conventional "referred" or "non-referred" groups. Such an assumption, if inaccurate, may contribute to discrepancies across studies in the nature and severity of emotional difficulties attributed to children during this highly stressful time. Furthermore, failure to check the comparability of such samples may rule out opportunities to identify, within the population of children of divorced parents, subgroups which would be useful targets of investigation in their own right.

The present study examines the adjustment of two groups of children of recently separated parents, one group whose parents had requested (but not yet received) divorce-related counseling, and a second group whose parents elected research participation only. The primary aims were to determine: (1) the extent to which the children approached "clinical" levels of maladjusted behavior, and (2) whether the children from those families requesting counseling were more maladjusted than children from families not requesting counseling at this time.

METHODS

Subjects

The total sample included 105 children, ages 4 to 16 years, whose families were participants in a study of the impact of divorce on children conducted in Philadelphia and the surrounding suburban areas. In all but a few cases, the mother had custody of the children. Roughly half the sample (N = 56) were children whose parents elected to receive counseling services for divorce-related issues

(Requestors), while the remaining families (N = 49) volunteered as research subjects only (Non-requestors). Families were solicited for participation in research via newspaper advertisements, public service announcements, and word-of-mouth contacts. Upon their initial call to the project, the families were asked if they were calling to request counseling or to participate in the research only. No child was admitted to the study who had a history of referral for mental health services, or any intellectual or organic impairment. Roughly equivalent numbers of boys and girls participated, although there were slightly fewer girls among Requestors; 33 boys and 23 girls were in the Requestors sample, and 22 boys and 27 girls in the Non-requestors sample. The age distribution over the two groups was also equivalent, with a mean age of 8.3 years for the total sample, and 8.6 and 8.0 years for Requestors and Non-requestors respectively. The racial composition of the two groups was virtually identical, with each sample comprising of 73% white, and 27% black. Both the Requestors and Non-requestors had been married on average 11 years at the time of the separation. For the entire sample, the length of time between the separation and the interview averaged seven months. The Non-requestors had been separated 8.3 months and the Requestors 5.8 months. Ninety-one per cent of the sample had been separated one year or less, with the remainder separated no more than twenty months.

Though generalizations to a larger divorcing population must remain tentative due to the sampling procedure, the sample nonetheless has several advantages over most previous divorce studies. First it is relatively large for a divorce study that involves in-depth interviewing; second, the children were screened for gross psychopathology so that we could examine the effects of the divorce experience on normal children; and third, the sample is varied with respect to demographic and status characteristics. Following the example of another longitudinal divorce study, we argue that "although the sample was not selected randomly, it is quite heterogeneous, reflecting the ethnic, religious, and socioeconomic diversity of the locale in study. In most respects it is probably a good approximation of the population at large. . . " (Furstenberg, 1981, p. 2).

Instrumentation

Recent developments in the assessment of childhood maladjustment have yielded numerous empirically-based measures that could efficiently supplement more qualitative or divorce-specific approaches (McDermott, 1982). One such instrument which is used in the present study, is the Child Behavior Checklist (Achenbach and Edelbrock, 1978a, 1979, 1981, 1983) which was designed to provide reliable and standardized means of evaluating children's problems and competencies on the basis of parent's observations. An extensive standardization sample, including both randomly-selected normal children and those from clinic populations, permits differential classification of individuals or groups according to empirically-derived behavioral norms. The present study uses the revised scoring method (Achenbach and Edelbrock, 1983).

The Child Behavior Checklist (CBCL) presents parents with 118 items describing problem behaviors found to occur with relative frequency among clinical groups and rarely in the population-at-large. The parent indicates the extent to which each behavior is characteristic of his/her child according to a three-point scale. It further presents parents with 20 items that tap social competence with respect to participation in a variety of typical childhood activities, such as chores, sports, and hobbies, as well as social relationships and academic performance. Following Achenbach and Edelbrock's (1983) method, the items were reduced to a total behavior problems scale and a social competency scale. One component of the social competency scale is a separate scale that measures school performance. These scales are based on standardized scores and each has an expected normal group mean of 50 and a standard deviation of 10. The recommended cut-off score for membership in a clinical group is 70 for the Behavior Problem scales, on which higher scores are associated with more symptomatic behavior, and 30 for the Social Competence and School indices, on which lower scores point to fewer adaptive skills. Thus Achenbach defines as clinical, those scores that are two or more standard deviations beyond the expected normal mean. Reported inter-rater and test-retest reliability coefficients are in the moderate to high range (.54 to .98), and the CBCL's validity for discriminating between normal and clinical groups has been established (Achenbach, 1978; Achenbach and Edelbrock, 1978a, 1979, 1981, 1983). While the present study is based on scores from only one parent, Achenbach and Edelbrock (1983) report that ratings by mothers and fathers are correlated .99 for the behavior problems and .98 for the social competence items.

Procedures

CBCL ratings were obtained from the mothers based on their observations of the child's behavior. Although ratings were obtained for all 4 to 16 year olds, only one child per family was included in this study to insure independence of observations. Where there was more than one child in the appropriate age range, ratings used were of the child identified by parents as experiencing the greater difficulty with the separation, or, if parents could not single out one sibling over others, the oldest child in the family. Because the age specifications for the behavior, social and school scales are somewhat different, the number of children for whom each scale was calculated varies.

Statistics

Means for the Behavior, Social and School Scales were calculated for the total sample and separately for the Requestor and Non-requestor groups. These observed means were then compared to Achenbach and Edelbrock's (1983) expected normal and clinical scores respectively. In order to test for statistically significant differences between the observed means and the expected normal mean of 50 and the clinical cut-off of 70, ninety-nine per cent confidence intervals were placed around the observed means. Additionally, we calculated the percentage of children falling within the clinical range of each scale. In order to compare the Requestor and Non-requestor groups, a one-way analysis of variance with covariates was performed for each scale. The age and sex of the child as well as the length of separation were introduced as covariates both to estimate their effects and to control for any differences between the groups with respect to these factors.

RESULTS

Table 1 summarizes the distributions of the Behavior Problems, Social Competence and School scores for the total sample which includes both the Requestors and Non-requestors. The mean Behavior Problem score is substantially above the expected normal mean of 50, while the means for both the Social Competence and School scores are below the expected normal mean. The reader is reminded that a greater degree of maladjustment is indicated by

Table 1: Summary statistics for Behavior Problems, Social Competence and School Scores for combined Requestor and Non-Requestor sample.

	Behavior:	Social:	School:
Mean:	59.09	41.34	44.42
Standard Deviation:	11.64	10.75	8.45
99% Confidence Interval:	56.81-61.37	39.06-43.62	42.32-46.52
Percent within clinical range:	18.1%	21.3%	7.7%
Number of Observations:	105	89	65

Notes: The expected normal mean for each scale is 50 with an expected standard deviation of 10. Higher scores indicate a greater degree of maladjustment for the Behavior Problems scale; scores 70 and above are within the clinical range. For the Social Competence and School scales, lower scores indicate a greater degree of maladjustment and scores 30 or below are in the clinical range (Achenbach & Edelbrock, 1983).

The number of observations varies across scales because of differences in the age specificity of each.

higher scores for the Behavior Problem scale and lower scores on both the Social Competence and School scales. For each of the three scales, the 99 percent confidence interval encompasses neither the expected normal mean of 50 nor the clinical cutoff score (70 for Behavior Problems; 30 for Social Competence and School scales). Thus, our sample as a whole falls between Achenbach and Edelbrock's (1983) normal and clinical standardization sample and is significantly different from both at the .01 level. About 20 percent of the children fell within the clinical range for both behavior problems and social competence, and about 8 percent fell within the clinical range for the school score.

Requestors and Non-requestors were considered separately in comparison to the normal and clinical standardization samples to explore potential differences in their relative contributions to the pattern that emerged when all subjects were taken together. Table 2

Table 2: Summary statistics for Behavior Problems, Social Competence and School Scores for the Requestor and Non-requestor samples.

REQUESTOR SAMPLE

	Behavior:	Social:	School:
Mean:	61.79	39.24	43.95
Standard Deviation:	11.86	11.51	9.15
99% Confidence Interval:	58.61-64.97	36.02-42.46	40.95-46.95
Percent within clinical range:	36.8%	33.3%	10.8%
Number of Observations:	56	51	37

NON-REQUESTOR SAMPLE

	Behavior:	Social:	School:
Mean:	56.00	44.16	45.04
Standard Deviation:	10.69	9.02	7.54
99% Confidence Interval:	52.94-59.06	41.24-47.08	42.18-47.90
Percent within clinical range:	8.2%	5.3%	3.6%
Number of Observations:	49	38	28

Notes: The expected normal mean for each scale is 50 with an expected standard deviation of 10. Higher scores indicate a greater degree of maladjustment for the Behavior Problems scale; scores 70 and above are within the clinical range. For the Social Competence and School scales, lower scores indicate a greater degree of maladjustment and scores 30 or below are in the clinical range (Achenbach & Edelbrock, 1983).

The number of observations varies across scales because of differences in the age specificity of each.

shows that for both Requestors and Non-requestors, mean scores on all three scales differ from both the expected normal means and the clinical cut-off scores at the .01 level of significance.

Thus, in this sample of children of recently separated parents, certain consistencies emerged whether the Requestors and Non-requestors were considered separately or together. Behavior Problem Scale means were roughly midway between the clinical cut-off score of 70 and the expected normal group mean of 50, and different from both to a statistically significant extent. For both Social Competence and School scales, a similar pattern emerged with scores falling between the clinical cut-off of 30 and the expected normal mean of 50.

Table 2 also illustrates substantial differences between the Requestors and Non-requestor groups. Those requesting counseling showed a greater degree of maladjustment in all three areas examined. This is reflected in both the mean scores and the percentage of each sample that fell within the clinical range. While fewer than ten percent of the Non-requestors fell in the clinical range for any of the three scales, more than one-third of the Requestors fell in the clinical range for both the Behavior Problem and Social Competence scales. The 99 percent confidence intervals indicate that the Requestors are significantly more maladjusted than the Non-requestors at the .01 level for these two scales. There was not a significant difference with regard to the school scale. Therefore we see that while each group is different from both the expected normal and clinical scores, they are also different from each other, with those requesting aid closer to the clinical cut-off than those not requesting aid.

In order to control for possible confounding effects, the differences between the Requestor and Non-requestor samples were tested while holding constant the length of separation and the age and sex of the children. Table 3 summarizes the results of a one-way analysis of variance for the Behavior Problem and Social Competence scales. None of the three control variables which were introduced as covariates had a significant effect. The main effects indicate the significant differences between the Requestor and Non-requestor samples persist even with age, sex and length of separation taken into account.

DISCUSSION

Taken together the findings of the present study support the results of prior research which have indicated the likelihood of

Table 3: Analysis of variance results testing differences between the Requestor and Non-requestor samples for the Behavior Problems scale and Social Competence scale, controlling for the length of separation and child's age and sex.

BEHAVIOR PROBLEMS SCALE

Source of Variation	F	DF	Significance
Covariates-			
Length of Separation	.85	1	.36
Child's Age	.91	1	.34
Child's Sex	1.30	1	.26
Main Effect-			
Requestor/Non-Requestor	6.43	1	.01**

Number of Observations= 105

SOCIAL COMPETENCE SCALE

Source of Variation	F	DF	Significance
Covariates-			
Length of Separation	.21	1	.65
Child's Age	.07	1	.80
Child's Sex	.49	1	.49
Main Effect-			
Requestor/Non-Requestor	5.67	1	.02*

Number of observations= 89

* significant at .05 level or less
** significant at .01 level or less

Note: The effects of the covariates were estimated first, followed by the main effects. In this manner, the effect of Requestor/Non-requestor status is ascertained holding constant the effects of the length of separation (in months) and the child's age and sex.

emotional or behavior problems for many children in the aftermath of parental separation (Hetherington et al., 1978; Hodges et al., 1979; Longfellow, 1979; Young and Parish, 1979). There was no indication, however, that clinical levels of disturbance predominated. Rather, there was a tendency for many children in the present study to show difficulties in social relations, and to display behavior indicative of distress to an intermediate extent; that is, more than would be expected in a randomly-chosen normal group, yet not to the degree characteristic of a clinically-disturbed population. These tendencies were obtained whether the sample was considered in aggregate, or broken down into subgroups of those who had requested and those who did not request aid.

While a substantial number of children fell into the "normal" range of the standardized scales, more qualitative approaches would almost certainly reveal problems and concerns among children of separating parents that are not detected by a standardized test. Standardized and qualitative measures are both important in obtaining a more complete picture of adjustment and may each provide different and equally valid information. Despite the limitation using standardized tests, it was noteworthy that a substantial number of children maintained a normal level of functioning on tests that distinguish disturbed from non-disturbed groups, especially in light of prevailing trends in the literature.

Comparisons between our two groups—those who requested and those who did not request counseling—calls to question assumptions in divorce research that children whose parents have sought divorce-related counseling are representative of all children of divorcing parents. Statistically significant differences between the two groups emerged on two of the three indices of adjustment with only school performance similar across the two groups. Children whose parents requested counseling were more likely than those in the non-counseling group to receive ratings that placed them towards the clinical extremes of maladjustment in terms of social competence and behavior problems. Despite considerable overlap between the two groups in the normal range of scores, this trend towards a higher incidence of adjustment problems among those requesting aid was sufficiently consistent and pronounced to suggest difficulties in generalizing findings drawn from a divorce counseling group to the general population of families of divorce. Those families requesting counseling are likely to include a higher percentage of children with marked emotional or behavioral problems than would be found in a more heterogeneous sample of divorcing families. It is noteworthy, however, that neither Requestors nor Non-requestors appeared representative of a clinical population and each is likely to be a distinct and important constituency in the study of children's response to divorce.

Unlike several previous studies, we did not find levels of adjustment to be related either to the child's age or sex. Those studies, however, examined a different age range or relied upon qualitative measures. Further research is needed on the possibility of age and sex differences across various dimensions of adjustment.

In conclusion, the use of a counseling sample alone is likely to limit the ability to generalize findings to a non-counseled sample. The present study has identified important differences between the children of families who have requested counseling and those that did not during the first year of the separation. The persistence of these differences over time is an empirical question that must be addressed through longitudinal research.

REFERENCES

Achenbach, T. M. (1978). Psychopathology of childhood: Research problems and issues. *Journal of Counseling and Clinical Psychology, 46*, 759–776.

Achenbach, T. M. and Edelbrock, C., (1978a). The child behavior profile: I, boys aged 6–11, *Journal of Counseling and Clinical Psychology, 46*, 478–488.

Achenbach, T. M. and Edelbrock, C. (1978b). The classification of childhood psychopathology: A review and analysis of empirical efforts. *Psychological Bulletin, 85*, 1275–1301.

Achenbach, T. M. and Edelbrock, C. (1979). The child behavior profile: II, boys aged 12–16 and girls aged 6–11 and 12–16. *Journal of Consulting and Clinical Psychology, 47*, 223–233.

Achenbach, T. M. and Edelbrock, C. (1981). Behavioral problems and competencies reported by parents of normal and disturbed children. *Monographs of the Society for Research in Child Development, 46*, Serial No. 188.

Achenbach, T. M. and Edelbrock, C. (1983). Manual for the child behavior checklist and revised child behavior profile. Queen City Printers, United States.

Dreger, R. M. (1981). First-, second-, and third-order factors from the child behavior classification project instrument and an attempt at rapprochement. *Journal of Abnormal Psychology, 90*, 242–260.

Furstenberg, F. F. (1981). Renegotiating parenthood after divorce and remarriage. Presented at the Society for Research in Child Development Symposium on Changing Family Patterns, Boston, MA.

Goetting, A. (1981). Divorce outcome secured. *Journal of Family Issues, 2*, 350–378.

Hetherington, E. M. (1972). Effects of father absence on personality development in adolescent daughters. *Developmental Psychology, 7*, 313–326.

Hetherington, E. M., Cox, M. and Cox R. (1978). The aftermath of divorce. In J. H. Stevens Jr. and M. Matthews (Eds.) *Mother/Child, Father/Child Relationships*, National Association for the Education of Young Children, Washington, D.C., 149–176.

Hodges, W. F., Wechsler, R. and Ballantine, C. (1979). Divorce and the preschool child: Cumulative stress. *Journal of Divorce, 3*, 55–67.

Holmes, T. H. and Rahe, R. H. (1967). The social readjustment rating scale. *Journal of Psychosomatic Research, 11*, 213–218.

Isaacs, M. B. (1985). Traversing The Experience Well: A Three Year Study of Divorce. Paper presented at the 62nd Annual Meeting of the American Orthopsychiatric Association, Inc., New York City, New York.

Kulka, R. A. and Weingarten, H. (1979). The long-term effects of parental divorce in childhood on adult adjustment. *Journal of Social Issues, 35*, (4): 50–78.

Longfellow, C. (1979). Divorce in context: Its impact on children. In G. Levinger and O. Moles (Eds.) *Divorce and Separation: Context, Causes and Consequences*, Basic Books, New York.

McDermott, J. F. (1968). Parental divorce in early childhood. *American Journal of Psychiatry, 23*, 421–427.

McDermott, J. F. (1971). Divorce and its psychiatric sequelae in children. *Archives of General Psychiatry, 23*, 421–427.

McDermott, P. A. (1982). The observation and classification of exceptional child behavior. In R.T. Brown and C.R. Reynolds (Eds.) *Psychological Perspective on Childhood Exceptionality*, Wiley and Son, New York.

Santrock, J. W., & Warshak, R. A. (1979). Father custody and social development in boys and girls. *Social Issues, 35*, 112–125.

Wallerstein, J. S. and Kelly, J. B. (1980). *Surviving the breakup: How Parents cope with divorce*. Basic Books, New York.

Young, E. R. and Parish, T. S. (1979). Impact of father absence during childhood on the psychological adjustment of college females. *Sex Roles, 3*, 217–227.

Children and Divorce: The "Negative" Identification

Morton Chethik
Nancy Dolin
Douglas Davies
Rebecca Lohr
Susan Darrow

In the growing literature on children and divorce, there is increasing attention directed toward the fate of the object tie of the child, since the child experiences a form of at least partial object loss (e.g., Chethik and Kalter, 1980; Tessman, 1978; Kelly and Wallerstein, 1974, 1976). What happens to the normal developmental process of identification when the parent leaves? What are the varied impacts at different age levels? Are identifications used "defensively" by the child in order to cope with loss? What occurs in the process of internalization within the child, if the divorcing parents polarize their own differences in personalities? These issues in identification have been an important focus of our study on "The Impact of Divorce on Children" for the last few years at the University of Michigan.

In our present paper, we wish to highlight one aspect of the problems in identification for these children, which we have termed the "negative identification." A strikingly common complaint many parents present about their child, at the point of referral and evaluation, is that their child is taking on the negative characteristics of the former spouse. Laments can be heard, like the following: "He is the spitting image of his father—stubborn, wild, impossible to control," or "living with his mother, he becomes more and more of a sissy, afraid even to go out and play," or "since his dad left several months ago, he acts more and more like his father. He is depressed and can sit for hours in his father's empty study. I don't

The authors are on the faculty and staff of the Department of Psychiatry, University of Michigan Medical School, 1402 Catherine Place, Ann Arbor, MI 48109.

know what to do.'' These negative descriptions of their youngsters are accompanied by a variety of affects: at times an empathic concern (what is happening to him since the divorce?); at times, by a helpless rage at the child who is making life miserable; or fury at the ex-husband whose ''bad influence'' on the children even extends years beyond the divorce. Since this is a rather common phenomena in the family of divorce, we have explored a large number of cases with this form of presenting complaint. We will present a number of these types of cases, discussing the variety of underlying meanings that have emerged, and some of the implications for intervention.

Initially, when confronted with this complaint, one must raise a critical question. Are there real changes—real shifts in identification within the child? If so, what is the impetus or motivation for the change? Or are we dealing primarily with a distorted perception of the child by a troubled parent? For example, does the parent misperceive certain characteristics within the child, and impute special meanings because of an underlying need to find some way to continue an old marital battle? In our experience, we have found many cases of real identificatory shifts within the child, following the divorce or separation, and on the other hand, many situations where projections by the parent act to distort the parent-child relationship. There are, as well situations where we see an interaction of both—some identification shifts within the child and intense reaction to the change by the parents. We will be discussing these varied aspects of the ''negative identification.''

IDENTIFICATION SHIFTS WITHIN THE CHILD: THE VARIED FUNCTIONS OF INTERNALIZATION

Identification is defined as a transformation of the self, whereby the self becomes similar to the external object. Schaffer (1968) notes that identification is an unconscious process, and, more precisely, that identification occurs when self-representation become like representations of the object. The process of identification, in normal development, is fostered in part by the natural daily separations from the object. Freud (1921) has noted that identification is a particular means of maintaining a close relationship to an object, and that it can be ''the sole condition under which the id can give up the objects.'' It is through identification that the child seeks to minimize his vulnerability to objects. We are all familiar with the beginning nursery school girl, who, when separated from home, begins to play "mommie" and "house" with the dolls and new girls around her. In the fantasy of her play, the mother and child are together, the anxiety about separation abates, and this is accomplished by an internalization of the functioning mother.

Clearly a similar process can occur when the growing child loses a parent through divorce. The identification with the parent can enhance the personality of the child by allowing him to preserve the relationship, and continue to make use of a mixture of affection and guidance given to him by that parent. The wholesome aspects of internalization come to our attention less than distorted or debilitating identifications. In our experience, the "negative" identificatory shifts within the child have invariably been used as defenses against the emergence of painful affects.

Internalization as a Defense Against Sadness (in Object Loss)

In our clinic, we have seen a significant number of children who are reacting to *acute* family disruption. They are referred to the clinic because symptoms and behavior changes quickly emerge, which often take the form of "negative identification" with the absent parent.

> Douglas (age 12), briefly noted above, was shattered by his father's sudden abandonment of the family. His father, a distinguished professor at a midwestern university, undergoing a mid-life crisis abruptly left his rather close unit family. Within two weeks of announcing his wish for a divorce, which came as a total surprise, he revealed he had had a long-term, serious relationship with another woman, moved out of the house, and relocated in a city 500 miles away. Douglas, a gifted youngster, had always shared his father's vigorous intellectual pursuits and the father had always enjoyed explaining complex phenomena in terms that his son could understand.
>
> In retrospect Douglas' mother had noted changes in her husband for the past few years—he was withdrawn, brooding and began to drink more heavily. When she had spoken with him, he described "work and career problems only."
>
> A significant aspect of the final departure of the father was

> the removal of all the professional books from the father's library. Douglas worked hard with his father, carefully packing and crating many boxes. The overt symptom picture that concerned the mother regarding Douglas was his growing isolation and increasing withdrawal, his affinity to sit in the empty study, and his halting speech which sounded too much like the speaking pattern of his father.
>
> As Douglas, in brief individual therapy, gave vent to his enormous sense of loss and desertion by his father the mirror identification abated. He slowly accepted and integrated the fact that his father was really away.

A number of children we see, who are struggling with the acute aspects of the loss, "become" the lost objects. This is usually a transient symptom picture, a partial identification, and a component of an acute grief process. It is difficult to define these identifications as true identifications where there is real change in the self. Rather these children, like Douglas, preserve the object through their action (mirroring behavior), but the behavior is still external to the subjective self. The behavior functions to keep the object alive, to maintain a sense of intimacy with the departing parent, until the child can better cope with the loss.

Internalization as a Defense Against the Anxiety of Helplessness

Another common variation of identification under severe stress is not due to the acute loss, but rather the intense and vivid pathology of the parting parent.

> Chip, age 9, was referred to the clinic by his mother who had been concerned about him since he was four. Her most immediate worry was Chip's very destructive behavior consisting of tearing up the house, breaking up furniture, and hitting or threatening her and himself. On a recent evening, when she had asked him to share a pillow with a visiting cousin he became intensely enraged, clenching his fists, turning red in the face, and threatening to throw a vacuum cleaner down the stairs at her. Then, with feelings of remorse and guilt, he threatened to stab himself. She stated that she was very fearful of what Chip might do to her or himself, and at those moments, "He looks exactly like his father." She and

Chip's father separated initially when Chip was 20 months of age, reconciled when he was three and divorced when he was six. On a number of occasions during those years, Chip witnessed his father totally demolish their house and belongings, along with more numerous episodes of abusing the mother. In the last and most frightening occurrence, the father smashed all of the furniture in Chips' bedroom, marked up the walls with black paint and left it uninhabitable. When Chip saw what happened, he said sadly, "Why did he do that to me? I didn't do anything to him."

The father had been diagnosed as a paranoid schizophrenic, and Chip's identification with his father had internal but also external reinforcements. Mother often felt she saw the father in Chip—they had the same "look in the eyes." Fearful of her own aggression, the mother provoked from her masochistic, passive position the aggressive attacks from husband and son, a reenaction of her experiences with her own alcoholic, abusive father. As this pathological and overdetermined identification was made conscious to the mother, she was better able to hold out different expectations for Chip's behavior and to experience less fear of his potential violence.

The major internal motivation for Chip to identify with his violent father was to cope with his fear through the mechanism of identification with the aggressor. As the tormentor, he was no longer in the fearful, passive victimized position he experienced as a young child.

The significant number of children we see identify with the characteristics of a lost, disturbed parent. They often, through their modelling, express the fear actively that they have the "bad genes" and will therefore share the same terrible fate (hospitalization, prison, suicide, illness) of the parent. Often these are identifications on an affect-motor level, ego alien to the child. Over time, however, they can become internalized self-representations.

Internalization as Fidelity—The Defense Against Abandonment

During the early years of life, as the child builds a coherent representation of the object, he at first splits off and separates the good and the bad aspects of the object. In early childhood the good "fairy godmother" stands in bold contrast to the bad "old witch" (actually the exaggerated good and bad aspects of the mother). A major task in development is, over time, to integrate the loving and frustrating aspects of the mother into a whole object, and build a realistic image of that object. Understandably the good aspects of the object are tenaciously held onto, since the child is totally dependent on his parents for survival. In a substantial number of children of divorce in our population, we note a fierce and dedicated loyalty to an absent parent, despite the actual objective negative, deserting or abusive characteristics of that parent. Often that loyalty is expressed in a "negative identification."

> Kathryn was 9 when she was brought to our clinic by her natural father and stepmother. Two issues were troubling to them. The characteristic of Kathy's lying which she resorted to consistently and pervasively was very disturbing. In addition was the poor relationship with the stepmother. Kathy persistently made a point of the separateness of the stepmother and herself—for example, loudly proclaiming to her class on the first day of school that Mrs. Q. was not her real mother, and refusing to take any handmade gifts home made at school for Mother's Day. After all, she said, she would not be seeing her mother.
>
> Kathryn had lived with her natural mother until she was five years of age, despite the father's attempt to gain custody. The mother was a very immature, inadequate woman, unable to provide for the needs of her daughter and finally deserted the child, running off with a new lover. Kathryn's natural mother was an ever present "ghost" in the new household, and her image caused intense feelings in the family members. The B's worried that Kathryn would turn out like her natural mother, who was a "pathological liar, irresponsible and promiscuous." In Kathryn's daily behavior, the evidence of this similarity seemed to accumulate.
>
> In therapy, Kathryn revealed the motivations for this mother-child identification. In her play a common theme was that desertion was always for virtuous reasons. In a special wolf family she used in her play, the mate left the family in order to find food or better shelter for the family. It was important to her wolf game that no one take over for the departed wolf while she was gone. Later in therapy she spoke directly and angrily about her vanished mother. "I am her

crutch: she leans on me. A person that needs a crutch can't walk without it.'' She explained that she could never abandon her natural mother, or ever come close to her stepmother. After all, she reasoned aloud—if she did not love her mother, who would? She could not bear the thought of her mother remaining alone and uncared for.

Only later in the therapy, her denial of the negative aspects of her mother abated. At one point, searching for some positive legacy about her mother, she asked her stepmother poignantly, ''Wasn't there anything good about my mother? The stepmother, sensing the internal emptiness and vulnerability to her daughter as she gave up the unreal image, helped her find some real assets—specific skills the mother had as a seamstress, etc.

Through the ''negative identification'' with the absent parent, a number of children continue to maintain the early mother-child aura of protection. Kathryn seeks to preserve the early mother-child union. It was clear that without the attachment to her real mother (even the failing mother), Kathryn felt that she herself was a vulnerable infant without a ''crutch'' and without anyone to love her in the world. This mother at times embodied the ''good fairy'' characteristics that protected her, despite the real neglect that occurred. The vulnerability of the past made her cling to the only form of protection she had during her early years.

Identification as Defense Against the Loss of Self-Esteem: Warding Off Threatening Aspects of the Self

Splitting,* as noted above, is a prominent mechanism used by children with an absent parent. Without the persistent frustrations inherent in the daily interactions which contain both rewards and frustrations, it is more difficult for the child to develop a realistic image of the parent. The absent parent can be idealized, and these idealizations are kept alive through self-representations. Often these characteristics serve important defensive functions.

---

*The term ''splitting'' is used descriptively to highlight particular problems in resolving ambivalence in children of divorce. This does not refer to the primitive form of ''splitting'' associated with borderline or narcissistically damaged children.

Jeremie, age 10, was referred because of his general depressed, but also ''hang-dog'' demeanor. Mother and stepfather noted that Jeremie was a ''sweet boy,'' good to everybody, ''wouldn't hurt a fly'' but somehow failing to do what other boys do. He wasn't competitive, interested in sports, etc. They described characteristics which troubled them. Jeremie was very protective of his mother (e.g., ''Are you all right mother?'', or ''I though you might be sick.''). He was also a special guardian of a neighborhood youngster who was severely scapegoated by peers, thereby alienating himself from the larger group of potential and more typical friends. The stepfather felt he was unable to ''influence'' Jeremie, felt pushed away by him, and there were times he was ''ready to throw in the towel.''

Jeremie's natural father left the family when he was three years old, but he maintained a weekly contact throughout the years. In gathering the history, mother felt that in addition to the divorce, another important event was her own ''emotional crisis.'' This occurred when Jeremie was two and lasted for two years. The mother became depressed, was emotionally labile and just ''went through the motions'' of raising her children. Despite the growing antipathy with her husband (and divorce in this period) the basic nurturance and care of the children fell to the natural father. He clearly took over for the mother, until she was able to function well. The father was a ''good, kind man.''

In the therapy with Jeremie he idealized the sensitive, caring father who had maintained the old family home. In contrast, as treatment unfolded, the outlines of a larger tyrannical, menacing male that threatened the helpless and weak became clear in play. A mean landlord who owned many houses, had to be fought by a little boy and his mother. A rich foreigner with vast oil holdings was taking advantage of a young woman who was at his mercy, since she needed shelter and clothing for her offspring. The real ''cruel'' stepfather came into open discussion, and he contained the repelling attributes of the phallic sexual man and the aggressive, acquisitive father. The good, nurturant father of pre-oedipal times (idealized, asexual, unaggressive and protective) was maintained through an identification, while Jeremie lived with all that was despised and feared. The function of the identification was to maintain a defensive splitting—if he could hold onto his idealized father, he could also ward off the oedipal features within himself.

Once the image of the cruel stepfather was consciously aired, it was hard to maintain it realistically. While the "mean" man gave out chores and yelled at times, he was also a good athlete who offered to teach Jeremie. He also had a striking capacity to buy little items that Jeremie needed. And the real father's image slowly became tarnished. Jeremie could not deny that his father had a consistent girl friend who slept over with him, and that father had recently missed weekend visits to be with her. Jeremie in turn began missing visits, and had dreams of his real father suffering heart attacks. His sexuality was also aroused—dreams of astronauts and policemen who performed heroic feats emerged. With a new group of male friends, he spoke excitedly of their secret fantasies of pulling bikinis off girls. The protective, subservient identification gave way to a more assertive, engaging style of relating.

The function of the "negative identification" was the maintenance of a special sense of self, and this was done in harmony with the idealized object. Jeremie also needed to markedly defend against the early rage toward his deserting father.

Anti-Identification—Another Defense Against Self-Esteem Loss

In a large number of the cases we have seen, the marriage (prior to divorce) has been marked by open resentment and contempt between mother and father. These divorcing parents often polarized and exaggerated their differences in specific personality characteristics. These "hated" characteristics symbolizing each parent were often sex linked—standing for "woman" or "man." For the child within the family, the characteristics of both parents are naturally internalized and some of these "devalued" qualities become hated characteristics associated with the self. We have seen a number of children attempting to extrude this "negative identification" by struggling to deny and push away these partially internalized qualities.

Adrienne, age 12, was referred six months after the parents' separation. She was an only child, and after the separation, mother and Adrienne moved to a new community 50 miles from the original home. Mother was most concerned about the explosive episodes between her and her daughter. Adrienne had frequent tantrums, called her mother "bitch," described how she hated her and blamed her totally for the divorce.

The K's marriage had always been a stormy one. Father was a successful businessman, a charming, engaging "wheeler dealer" who like to have his own way. Throughout the marriage there was often a battle of wills. Mother was vocally upset with father's possible unfaithfulness. Father expressed contempt about mother's general weaknesses. She was not, he felt, a firm or effective disciplinarian with Adrienne. She was always weak and giving. He also contemptuously described her lack of logic and complete emotionality. She was always "getting upset" and if not careful, he often baited her with the idea that she would have a nervous breakdown and end up in the hospital. Clearly, for Adrienne, vulnerability and expressing one's upset feelings were linked with being feminine.

During the early phases of treatment, Adrienne completely derided anything that was womanly in herself. Her dress and manner reflected the Tomboy. She preferred to hunt and shoot with her grandfather over anything else. She enjoyed coed sking but always ended up on the tougher hills with boys alone. She took great pleasure in stories and action where she was naughty, mischievious and defiant—tough characteristics thought to be admired by father. She couldn't stand the cheerleader types at school who used makeup and acted real flirty with boys. Her contempt for her mother mirrored her father's attitude. In her sessions she quoted her mother with sarcasm in their battles. "Stop it Adrienne, I'm not feeling well. If you don't stop, I'll end up in the hospital."

As treatment progressed, a major area of work centered on Adrienne's memories of the bitter fights between mother and father. The therapist interpreted and worked through Adrienne's enormous wish to please and be accepted by her father, and how that seemed to entail pushing away her womanly feelings. Some hidden femininity could then emerge. Slowly Adrienne described her crushes since first grade, and her current romantic feelings toward Tom, a boy in her class. There was a growing attraction and identification with her "female psychiatrist." She became interested in clothing, shoes and crossing her legs like her therapist. The femininity of her therapist was safer than that of her mother. The fear of identification was only one major factor in Adrienne's conflict with her mother. She also feared the underlying dependency strivings of her mother, and fought them by attempting to alienate her mother totally.

A number of our patients need to consciously reject the characteristics of the "hated" same sex parent, with whom they have begun to identify. They attempt to deny any resemblance to this devalued external object by adopting characteristics which are in direct opposition to the qualities of that parent. A major underlying motive is the fear that should the identification become evident, they would risk being rejected and extruded by the parent of the opposite sex. In this general situation the concept of the "negative identification" becomes an important dynamic within the child, and a force of anti-identification.

THE ROLE OF THE PARENT IN THE "NEGATIVE IDENTIFICATION" PROCESS

In our discussion thus far we have focused on a number of factors we have described *within* the child which can promote the "negative identification"—e.g., coping with acute loss, expressions of loyalty to the lost parent, etc. It has also been clear in our population that for a significant number of these children the parents make a major contribution in developing the perceptions of a "negative identification" within the child. In these cases, external issues within the family are highly significant. A major part of our intervention must then focus on the parent and his needs to distort or markedly reinforce a disturbed image of the child. We have noted in many of our families that with a father out of the home, the mother unconsciously pushes the child to take complementarity to a neurotic conflict.

The Parental Need to Reestablish Previous Marital Balances

Jeff, age 2-1/2, was seen with his mother in once weekly conjoint treatment for seven months.

During the evaluation, Mrs. T said that Jeff was unmanageable. When she tried to discipline him, he would respond by kicking or hitting her. He was also aggressive at his day care center. Jeff was a little tough guy: he never cried, and when he got hurt, he pretended not to be. Prior to his parents' separation when he was two, Jeff had seen his father beat up his mother several times and had been present during many arguments. Mrs. T described her husband as violent and unstable. After describing her husband's apparently severe characterological problems, she said, "I can see it all in Jeff. He looks like his father." During the marriage she had tried, by being kind and supportive, to reform her husband; now she sought treatment to "reform" her son.

During the first interview (in which both Mrs. T and Jeff were present), Mrs. T described her husband's violence, including an incident, when Jeff was two, when Mr. T had shattered the glass of the front door, showering Mrs. T and Jeff, who was in her arms, with broken glass. Jeff had screamed and began hitting his mother, which she understood as his anger towards her for having refused to let his father in. As she finished the story, Jeff lowered a roaring dinosaur into a baby's crib, saying "Monster bite baby." In the next hour, the monster repeatedly broke down a door to bite the baby and the baby's mother. The therapist suggested to Mrs. T that Jeff had experienced his father as a terrifying monster. His aggressive attacks were his attempt to master his fear by becoming the aggressor himself.

However, Mrs. T continued to complain of Jeff's aggression towards her at home. When he hit her, she would tell him how sad she felt. She did not feel restraining him would do any good. She described herself as a passive person who felt at the mercy of others' whims, but who hoped nevertheless that her kindness and gentleness would influence them to become kind and gentle themselves. She admitted that this strategy had not worked with her husband. It was evident that she was unable to give up her husband. Even though he had left the state and no longer contacted her, she had been unable to complete the divorce procedures. Her passivity in the fact of her little boy's aggression betrayed an unconscious wish to perpetuate her sadomasochistic relationship with her husband. As long as she responded to Jeff in terms of this relationship, she could not offer him the protection, firmness and empathy he needed.

Mrs. T was resistant to the therapist's initial attempts to explore this unconscious side of her relationship with Jeff. She continued to emphasize how much Jeff was like his father.

However, the therapist was able to make use of a strong treatment alliance to encourage Mrs. T to assure Jeff that she intended to protect him. These assurances, combined with interpretations specifying the origins of his fears in scenes of his father's violence, led to a lessening of symptoms at nursery school, though he remained aggressive towards his mother.

In a decisive hour during this period, Jeff pretended to pour scalding coffee on his mother's leg. When she pretended to feel sad, he picked up a lincoln log and began hitting her hard on the leg. She showed her pain, but did not resist or stop him. The therapist took the log from Jeff, telling him that he would not let him hurt his mother, nor would he hurt him. Jeff struggled for a moment and then looked very frightened. His mother took him on her lap and comforted him.

The following week Mrs. T said she had realized that she had reacted to Jeff's aggression just as she had to her husband's. The therapist noted that Jeff must have been extremely frightened when he witnessed her vulnerability and passivity when his father had attacked her. He must have felt that he too could become the object of his father's beatings, and that she would be unable to protect him. He had resolved this dilemma by becoming like his father. Now, when he sensed vulnerability in his mother, he would become aggressive towards her. Her response of not protecting herself would scare him even more, further fueling his aggression. Mrs. T agreed, saying she realized she was making it worse for Jeff by being passive and pretending to cry. The therapist said that when he had restrained him, Jeff had shown us that beneath the impervious tough guy was a frightened little boy.

Once the negative identification was broken, Mrs. T could empathize with Jeff's fears and began to take on a firm parenting role with him. During the next month she reported success in restraining his attacks and in talking with him about his worries. Her firmness allowed him to relax his alert, aggressive defense, so that he felt less need to become a threatening man in order to feel safe.

Mrs. T's acknowledgement of her chosen role as passive victim led to limited exploration of the roots of this style, and to considerable working through of her ambivalent relationship with her husband. Slowly she gave him up, a process that was marked concretely when she took the necessary legal steps to finalize the divorce. Jeff's own working through involved much pretending to be hurt and his mother's firm assurances that she would protect him.

In this case, when Mrs. T was able to stop seeing Jeff in the image of her husband and to become a protective parent, Jeff in turn could begin to give up his defensive identification with his violent father.

The Parental Need to Continue to Reactiviate Early Childhood Conflicts

We have found in many of our cases that the child in the family of divorce often carries a distorted, unconscious meaning for the parent. This stems from repressed conflicts from within the original family. (This is, of course, true for children in families where there is no divorce, as well.) Children can come to represent unacceptable aspects of the self, or a specific troubling member of the primary family. The child can also unconsciously arouse the difficult past parent-child union, or foster a frightening ''return'' of early repressed family trauma. A particular variation in which the ''negative identification'' clearly emerges is when the former spouse carried specific distorted projections which become transferred to the child following the divorce.

Mrs. R was an attractive woman in her early thirties, who was markedly upset by rather chronic problems with her six year old son, David. She had been divorced several years earlier (final separation occurred when David was 3-1/2 years of age), and she was now completing her credits toward a graduate degree.

She expressed a lot of concern about the fighting relationship she had with David. She found she was furious with him almost all of the time, and he fought back. He would not accept her authority—eating, dressing, etc. He was very stubborn and ended up saying, ''I won't.'' Since she was bigger, mother noted, she won and subdued him with force. She hated that they descended into that.

David embarrassed her a great deal. He had temper tantrums with the children of her friends, and he was extremely bossy and controlling of all of his friends. This controlling attitude, this "pushiness and domination" reminded her of her former husband whom she feared he would end up resembling. She felt he was clearly headed in that direction. Father and son liked to visit each other, and David never had trouble with his father.

Mrs. R also described her past marriage. Her husband was a very successful scientist in a large corporation. She admired her husband, but never loved him. He was an outstanding researcher, dynamic and hard driving. They could not talk to each other however, and the more competent her husband was, the less adequate she felt as a person. Even in child rearing, Mr. R was very effective and competent with David during his infancy and early years, and she had the feeling he was showing her up.

When she described her own history, she recalled a very unhappy childhood. Her parents separated and divorced when she was eleven. No one seemed to care about her. She recalled trying to "disappear into the woodwork" so no one would notice her. Her mother told her she was her "accident," and her father's concern was that she would become a financial burden on him. She recalled additionally being very competitive with a brother 16 months younger than herself.

While David was seen directly, mother also worked with David's therapist on the troubling aspects of her relationship with her son. At first she complained bitterly about her son's constant provocative behavior with her, which invariably led to their battles. After several months of work Mrs. R felt a measure of success when she could anticipate and step back from their confrontations. David responded somewhat with relief and good feeling.

In some sessions after one-half year of work, Mrs. R nostalgically recalled her pregnancy. She had a tremendous wish for a child. She had never been happier, and her husband had been attentive and loving. The first year with David had gone extremely well. She loved how he looked reposed in a crib and bassinet and she brought in a lock of his fine "baby" blond hair she had saved. Things changed in David's second year as the marriage deteriorated.

Mrs. R had a significant dream in this period. David as a

> toddler was alone in the kitchen in a high chair. There is only a picture of a man in the corner and she realized the picture was taking care of David. David fell in the dream, and Mrs. R awakened abruptly. In the session she wept intensely that she wasn't there for her son. She associated to her father who had never been there for her. The therapist noted that when David became an active toddler, that she felt she lost something very special. She was furious with David for going away from her and needing her less. This marked a change in their relationship. Mrs. R affectively felt some of her early attachment with David and "forgave him for growing up." A process of reciprocal affection began.
>
> Similar themes continue later in therapy. Mrs. R complained bitterly about David's restaurant behavior. He was "loud and dominating." As we followed the details, he caught the eye of the waitress, made sure he got a glass of water and a straw, talked directly to the busboy. Everyone at the restaurant, on appraisal, came to like David—but it made mother very uncomfortable.
>
> Some of David's "demandingness" emerged as interesting behavior. David asked a lot of questions and had many ideas. David, for example, questioned why he should only be allowed to play upstairs. He argued it was his house also, so mother should let him play elsewhere. When David put up his arguments, Mrs. R reacted with either helplessness or rage.
>
> As Mrs. R examined some her reactions, she described how she could not understand someone who wasn't shy or wasn't neat. A great deal of material emerged about her intense wish that David would have been a girl, someone like herself who she would have been comfortable with. David had the genes of her husband. He was afraid of nothing. Throughout the rest of the work with the mother, the therapist helped Mrs. R separate real problematic behavior from the energy of a robust phallic-oedipal boy.

Due to early deprivation in childhood, Mrs. R felt intensely that she was an inadequate person (an inadequate woman), envious of the world of all men. While she "admired" her successful husband, she couldn't love him; and in a similar way, she became conflicted about the activity and adequacy of her son. Mr. R's competence and David's outgoingness highlighted the mother's internal sense of her own damage. The mother's ''negative identification'' of both son and husband stemmed from intense feelings of competition from her own early childhood.

SUMMARY

In summary, in our experience, the process of the identification can often be used by the child as a defense, to cope with the affects stimulated by object loss. The affects evoked by divorce within the child are feelings of sadness, fears of abandonment, rage, loss of self-esteem (sense of worthlessness), and at times the anxiety provoked by these affects are warded off by a ''negative identification.''

Often these identifications are used as stop-gap measures and temporary devices to cope with the acute emergence of intolerable feelings. However, it is clear that in a significant number of cases, these seemingly transient internalizations harden into long-term characterological problems.

There appears to be two major conditions that help to solidify these identifications within the child. Internally, if the child continues to be unable to deal with the ''unacceptable'' affects, he will continue to maintain the defensive identification. Externally, if there is a strong parental need to ''see'' and reinforce these characteristics within the child, these identifications will become solidified.

While we have limited our discussion of the problem of ''negative identification'' to children of divorce, it is clear that other family situations can provoke similar problems within the child. Since these problems of identification will rise when parents are in conflict (when specific parental characteristics are degraded and devalued), children who grow up in families of the ''bad marriage'' can certainly have similar problems.

REFERENCES

Chethik, M. and Kalter, N. (1980). Developmental arrest following divorce: the role of therapist as developmental facilitator. *J Am Acad Child Psychiatry 19*, (2); 281–289.

Freud, S. (1921). Group Psychology and the Analysis of the Ego. SE 18. Hogarth Press, London.

Kelly, J.B. and Wallerstein, J.S. (1976). The effects of parental divorce. *Am J Orthopsychiatry 46*; 20–32.

Tessman, L. (1978). Children of Parting Parents. Aronson, New York.
Wallerstein, J.S. and Kelly, J.B. (1974). The effects of parental divorce. In Child and His Family, E.J. Anthony and C. Kapernik, eds., Wiley, New York, 479–505.
Wallerstein, J.S. and Kelly, J.B. (1975). The effects of parental divorce. *J Am Acad Child Psychiatry 14*; 600–616.

DEVELOPMENTAL FEATURES IN CHILDREN OF DIVORCE

"Where Is My Daddy's House?" Preschool-Age Children of Divorce and Transitional Phenomena – A Study

Ruth Stirtzinger

ABSTRACT. Preschool-age children of divorce not living in the family home show specific discrete longing for it. After divorce the family home may allow the preschool-age child the necessary mental image of access to both his parents – "transitional representation" at a time of decreasing family structure.

The literature over the last 10 years has begun to identify the effect of divorce on children. Some results stand out quite convincingly: (1) all children are affected by divorce regardless of age or the

Ruth Stirtzinger, MD, MA, FRCP(C), Faculty of the University of Toronto, Department of Psychiatry, and staff psychiatrist, Clarke Institute of Psychiatry, Family and Child Studies Centre, 250 College Street, Toronto MJT 1R8, Canada.

This pilot study paper was presented at the Scientific Meeting of the *American Academy of Child Psychiatry*, October 1984, Toronto, Canada.

quality of the relationship with their parents; (2) children of different ages show some specific and predictable reactions because of their age; (3) many parents prepare children little for this change in their life and the younger the child, the less preparation parents feel necessary to do.

This pilot study presents a new finding: preschool-age children undergoing the stress of their parents divorce show specific discrete longing for the family home. Mourning this object loss may strongly affect their adjustment to the divorce.

This work investigating preschool-age children, a group strongly affected by divorce, examines their thinking through art drawings and stories. In addition to a child's feeling of decreased dependability in primary relationships, this work shows that children no longer living in the family home display very different thought content and longings compared with children of divorce who still live in the family home.

Spontaneous drawings showed those children no longer living in the family home to be preoccupied with thoughts of the home. In contrast, the second group, living in the family home, focused not on the home but on their parents, featuring anxiety specifically with regard to the parents' existence: where they were, were they real, were they together. No differences were found as to whether the child lived with mother or father. The two groups were matched for age, socio-economic level, and absence of family pathology before the divorce.

This finding may not have been identified previously because (1) at the beginning of this last decade children more often stayed in the family home, with mothers not being financially able to leave and take the children with them, and (2) fathers were not as frequently acting as caretakers so that if he left the marriage and home he would leave the children in the family house with mother. Thus, children would have been taken from the family home less often.

These findings are related to Winnicott's transitional phenomena work, specifically hypothesizing the family home to be an intermediate territory between inner psychic reality and the external world. Like other transitional phenomena, the process represents a gradual decathection at the child's own pace as his internal representations solidify. The abrupt removal of this important object through separation and divorce ruptures the sequence of the developing object relations between child and his primary caretakers.

Evidence seen in the first group's drawings suggests that a child's mourning is fixated for a time at least around loss of the home and cannot proceed as quickly to the loss of the real parent objects or toward the process of seeing the parents as real people and adjusting to a new style of living.

The findings are also related to preschool-age children's intellectual development regarding their use of transductive and juxtaposition reasoning. The first mode of thinking, causing the young child to link together two unrelated pieces of information, may lead him to reason that if the family home is gone, parents may be gone too. Juxtaposition reasoning, concentrating on parts of an object and not relating the parts to the whole, or grasping the underlying concept, may cause belief that if the family home is gone, Mom and Dad are gone in some equally fundamental way.

Need for further study will be emphasized to define more explicit implications of the family home in the child's behavior after divorce and the style of defense mechanisms he uses in regard to the loss. This should be compared to the reactions of preschool-age children of nondivorced families moving from their home. Assessment tools should be increased and further include adjustment measures to compare the effect of living in the family home with being separated from it when a family divorces.

Implications of this study are explored as they relate to parents and health workers caring for children through divorce: i.e., allowing for a smoother transition from the family home; developing a construction of meaningful part objects from the home to be established in the child's new living environment; aiding the process of generalizing feelings from one physical space to another, legal policy regarding allocation of the family home may be affected.

METHOD

Subjects

Subjects were 8 preschool age children (3-1/2 to 6 years) whose parents had been separated or divorced for a period of 2 to 12 months. The term preschool is used here to designate the age group between the toddler period of development and school age years. Screening interviews took place to rule out clinical pathology in the families or developmental abnormalities in the children. The families were matched for socio-economic levels using the "Blishen Index" (1978). The children all attended a regular day care or nursery school. The subjects formed 2 groups, each consisting of 4 children; one group lived, currently, in the family home, the other group lived elsewhere and all lived with a custodial parent with open access to the other parent. All children lived with the mother except one from the first group.

Procedure

Data were gathered by holding two, two-hour long interviews with each group, inviting the children to draw or tell stories about whatever they wished. Care was taken not to introduce any topics but to elicit the child's own thought content.

The therapist was present to assist with needs like toileting and acquiring materials to record their stories and to gain objective information about the parenting.

Confidentiality was stressed to the children by the therapist's stating that their work was just "between the people in the room" and would remain there. They received special "star calendars" to take home with them after each session.

RESULTS

The results are summarized in Table 1. Over half of the pictures of group A were of houses with nearly one-half of these drawings representing the family house pictures. A story sample which accompanied one of these house drawings from a child not living in the family home stated: "The house has 2 bedrooms, a kitchen and a living room. The rooms are empty—no one lives there. A snake used to live there but she left because *they* didn't like the food. They all went away except the little tiny worm who stayed until she found her way home. One of *them* ate all the food—I'm going to get the bottle." Almost half of group B pictures were Mom and Dad together and 25% of group B were house pictures—half of these featured both parents in the house together.

In contrast nearly one-half of the group B pictures were of Mom and Dad together. Only one-quarter of these were of houses with one-half featuring both parents in the house together.

Table 1

Numbers and type of spontaneous picture drawings

GROUP A - WHO DO NOT LIVE IN FAMILY HOME	
Picture Content	Number of Picture Responses
The family house they were not living in	4/10
The present home with mention of the other home	2/10
A house	1/10
People - parent lived with	1/10
Other material	1/10

GROUP B - WHO LIVE IN FAMILY HOME	
Picture Content	Number of Picture Responses
Pictures of Mom and Dad together	6/16
A house	4/16
Picture of whole family	2/16
Parents	2/16
Self picture	1/16
A person picture	1/16

LITERATURE REVIEW AND DISCUSSION

Children's first recognizable drawings are of people—nothing is as interesting to children as the human face. Their drawings are coloured by feeling; they draw some but not all of what is known about the object; the drawings represent the child's inner realism and not the object reality. Children in both groups of the study drew proportionately more houses than would be expected when compared with general findings of children's drawings. The literature reports that children draw what is important to them; predominantly people, followed in frequency by animals, houses, and trees.

As early as 1885, in Italy, Ricci commented that young children drew what they knew existed and not what was actually seen. Prudhommeau, in France, stated that the child does not draw the object as it is but draws his idea of it—his "modele interne." Wolfe, in the U.S., noted that children's art refers to an inner realism, with emotions influencing the child's concept and drawings. Others agreed that the child's drawings represented intellectual and emotional elements. Piaget (1965) notes that the young child's reality is of his own mental construction; the child's vision is formed by his ideas.

The frequent drawing of houses in this study and, often, the house the whole family lived in designates the house as having great importance for these children. It leads one to speculate that the house has more importance for preschool age children of divorce than preschool children of intact families and that its taking precedence over drawing people and animals may imply its being given special symbolic meaning by these children.

While the present results are those of a pilot study with a small number of children, they need to be repeated with large numbers and compared to children of nondivorced families. We know that children draw people and live animals more than inanimate objects, yet in this pilot study the children of divorce, living in the family home were much more intent on object drawings than people drawings. Further, children of divorce not living in the family home drew houses or the family home more than twice as often as did the children of divorce living in the family home.

Why this preoccupation with the family home? Consider these examples:

1. A pediatrician reports on a 7-1/2 year old girl who is doing poorly at school, crying easily, having difficulty sleeping and not able to make friends since her parents' separation. He writes: "In speaking to Nicole, alone, it is clear that parental separation is creating a lot of concern on her part and it has been difficult to resolve. She does not feel she caused the split but does wonder if her parents will get back together again—she cries herself to sleep at night. It is interesting that her wish

was to move back to the family home rather than directly hoping that her parents will resolve their differences.''

2. A 3-1/2 year old, preparing to leave the family home with her mother due to parental separation, anxiously and repeatedly asks her mother ''Who gets my house? Who gets my toys? I take my toys outside and play with my friends. They take them in their house and keep them—who gets my house?''

It would seem a reasonable hypothesis that the family home is sought with increased intensity as is the transitional object or phenomena when certain potential conditions are present: when a caretaker is not present for a child; or in periods of regression, i.e., bedtime (Isaacs-Elmhurst, 1980). At such a time, a transitional object is often sought in preference to mother as a kind of idealized representation of her. Research shows that all children of all ages show some degree of regression post divorce (Hetherington and Cox, 1977; Wallerstein and Kelly et al., 1976).

Children of divorce appear to cling to the family home since the parents are not present in the usual way. C.J. Litt (1981) has shown that children who sleep with other family members have less use of a transitional object at night. Passman (1977), studying American children, showed blanket-attached children more able to overcome anxiety in a novel situation than those without attachment objects. Children of divorce may frequently call up images of the family home and, thereby, what it represents, to ward off the anxiety created from the disruption of their life by parental separation. It is akin to attachment behavior, seeking proximity to a love object, in this case, representation of a love object—the parents.

Passman (1976) reported that within the presence of the attachment object normal children showed: (1) increased exploratory behaviour and (2) facilitation of new learning. Is this mechanism of concentration on the family home used to allow children the security and stability they need to continue developing autonomous ego functions during a time of crisis?

Children at 2 months post divorce showed more non-functional play (that is repetitious muscle movements) and less imaginative play in all categories, than those of nondivorced families. Play is shorter and also contains less associative and co-operative features. Similarly, Hetherington and Cox (1979) have shown that the fantasy play present in children of divorce at all ages reveals an increase in imaginative play involving objects, namely, functional changes in objects and object related animation. Conversely, children of the same ages from nondivorced families spend more time interacting with imaginary people than objects. This may help explain the difference seen in the two groups in this study regarding the number of drawings related to objects rather than people.

Group B, who lived in a family home, demonstrated over half of their drawings to be primarily people pictures with almost half featuring Mom and Dad together. Twenty-five percent were object pictures—mainly house drawings.

Group A, who did not live in a family house, showed only between 10–20% people pictures with over half being object house pictures and almost half of those, old family house pictures.

Living in the family house or some close proximity to it may allow the child the necessary mental image of access to both his parents, i.e., a transitional representation at a time of changing family structure. He is more able to continue at normal developmental levels with this image.

Imaginativeness is an important feature in a child's play (Greenacre, 1959; Winnicott, 1971). Children who show spontaneous imaginativeness in play are likely to show a broader range of emotions and more positive affect than less imaginative children. Imaginative play is associated with self-control, low impulsivity and low aggression and with sharing, cooperation, independence and social maturity (Singer, 1976, 1977). Singer states "Imaginative play can be viewed as a major resource by which children can cope immediately with the cognitive, affective and social demands of growing up. It is more than a reactive behaviour, however, for it provides a practice ground for organizing new schemes and for transforming and storing material for more effective later expression in plans, actions or verbalization." This practice ground and intermediate territory between inner and outer realism is a vital area of growth and adjustment in life. That this illusionary area is necessary for mature development is essential to Winnicott's work in transitional object and phenomena theory (Winnicott, 1953; Hong, 1976; Bush, 1979).

Is the child who is undergoing parental separation using the family home as an intermediate territory to aid him in understanding and adjusting to the changes of his life and the changes in accessibility to his parents? Does it help him hold the mental image of having both his parents at a time when the internal reality of their physical separation threatens this?

Wallerstein and Kelly (1975), studying preschool age children at play after their parents' separation reported observing burdened, constricted, joyless play. The play was further characterized by aimlessness, wandering, desperate searching, and trying to fit objects together.

One child in this pilot study, 6 months after separation, each night desperately and compulsively drew many pictures of the family home, indeed, outlined the home several times on each picture. This could be seen as searching behavior and, as such, is akin to young children at rapprochement periods, who temporarily lose their parental object. As the child at rapprochement is aided by "the blanket," therapists may aid these children, whose parents have separated, by giving more attention to the transitional phenomena significant to them.

Could the family home or representations of it provide the media for the child to store memories of past love and at the same time develop and organize schema to contain the new ways he will now experience his parents? The family home, then, is conceived as being an intermediate territory between inner psychic reality and the external world. Like other transitional phenomena, it asserts a demand to be gradually decathected at the child's own pace, as his internal representations solidify. Separation/divorce, when it causes the abrupt removal of this important object, thus ruptures the sequence of the developing object relations between the child and his primary caretakers, especially when there are the superimposed changes in parental access that divorce entails. It does not allow gradual diffusion of transitional objects and their ultimate creation of symbolic play, which is still needed and enjoyed in adulthood. It may also be, from evidence seen in Group A's drawings, that the children's mourning is fixated for a time, at least, around loss of the home and cannot proceed as quickly to loss of the real parent objects or toward the process of seeing the parents as real people. Perhaps premature loss of this transitional object, which offers "idealism" at a time when it is needed causes increased defenses against the loss, in the form of retreating further from reality and so, at the same time, being even more threatened by it.

If this knowledge is used practically for children of divorce, attention to the family home or part objects representing it should be applied as soon as separation occurs. As seen in transitional object theory, in the prolonged absence of mother, the transitional object loses capacity to soothe (Ainsworth, 1963; Busch, 1974; Hong,

1976; Winnicott, 1953). It is in the immediate temporary absence of parental object that the transitional object is turned to.

Wallerstein and Kelly (1974) reported that the period immediately following separation seemed particularly useful in terms of effectiveness of intervention efforts. However, they also found that 80% of parents told children nothing, neither explaining the decision of the divorce nor of its even taking place—especially to preschool age children (Wallerstein and Kelly, 1980). Apparently divorcing parents are struggling with issues between one another at this time and tend to lose sight of the child's psychological needs because of their own turmoil.

It is possible that identifying these issues with parents, such as how the child will prepare to leave the family home, will draw their attention to the child and identify what is happening, so that it cannot be as easily disregarded. The home, the child's attachment to it, what it represents to him, can be a temporary concrete focus through which the parents may communicate with the child about changes taking place.

The preschool age child's intellectual developmental stage may also explain some of his preoccupations with the family home at this time. In a very fundamental way, he has difficulty cognitively separating it from his parents whom he knew and experienced there. Transductive reasoning in the preoperational stage of intellectual development in the preschool age child, as described by Piaget, affects the child's connecting his family home to the continuation of his relationship with his parents.

Piaget reports his daughter Jacqueline's conversation when she was ill and requested oranges. Piaget told that her oranges were still green and not yet ripe. Later, as Jacqueline drank her camomile tea, she said, "Camomile isn't green, it's yellow already . . . Give me some oranges." The child's reasoning made sense to her. If tea is yellow, then oranges must be yellow at this time too. Jacqueline attempted to link two separate bits of information together and the result was faulty prelogical reasoning.

It is possible to see how the young child would think that with the family home gone, Mom and Dad may be gone too, since they seemed to be so closely linked with the family home. Divorce literature reports that children, post separation, doubt the stability of relationships. Wallerstein and Kelly (1975) reported a shaken view of relationship dependability. In this study, similarly, the children asked "Who is my real Mom"? and "Will my Daddy find another little boy"?

Juxtaposition reasoning, another aspect of preoperational children's thinking patterns, concentrates on details and part of an object and does not relate the parts to the whole. The family house is gone—Mom and Dad are gone in some equally fundamental way. Likewise, living in the family home may cause the child to resist seeing the new routine of his parents' life. "If the home is the same then parent's life is the same." "If the home is gone, then his parents are gone" may be the reasoning for the preschool age child. The whole underlying the concept of them still being his parents and he their child, is seen with some difficulty. This may offer some explanation for the large number of "Mom and Dad" together pictures from the group living in the family home, and the dearth of them from the other group.

What can be done? Awareness of this kind of preschooler's thinking process, of the role the family home plays in his emotional security, whether the child lives in the family home or not, can aid the parent and therapist to understand the child's confusion after divorce. There are frequent findings that boys and girls several years after divorce still long for their parents to reunite and spend considerable energy on this wish (Hetherington and Cox 1978). Concrete object representation of the family home or of Mom's home and Dad's home may aid the child in mentally separating his old home from his new one, and in separating the fact of Mom and Dad not living in the family home from the fact that they are still his parents and care for him.

It seems that a variety of reactions could occur from either living in the family home or being separated from it.

Living in the family home may allow the preschool-age child to:

1. be more able to see himself as still having both parents because of close proximity to (still living in) the family home and thereby have the representational mental image of the family.
2. cling to the false idea that the divorce has not occurred and resist the changes in life style necessary.
3. deal more directly with people loss rather than the representation of loss—the family home.

These initial findings give impetus to future studies with a larger sample of children. Such studies might consider the following hypotheses:

1. The abrupt removal of the family home, when the family is separating or divorcing causes a significant increase in the developing relationships between the child and his primary caretakers, at a time when is he already feeling decreased dependability on parents because of their divorce. This would cause decreased developmental adjustment in children who are already experiencing a family crisis.
2. Children not living in the family home have their mourning fixated, at least for a time, around loss of the home and cannot proceed as quickly to adjust to the loss of real parent objects or toward the process of seeing the parents as real people and adjusting to a new lifestyle.

Future study, as well as examining the children's though content and process through structured play interviews, stories and drawings, should include standardized scales to measure developmental adjustment in children.

A control group—preschool age children of non-divorced families moving from their family home—should be added and examined with the same measures and at similar time intervals as the other two target groups.

The study has implications for parents and health care workers caring for children through the divorce. If the hypothesis of the family home taking on new meaning and affecting the child's adjustment is proven valid in further study, it may influence:

1. efforts at effecting a smoother transition from the family home.
2. developing representations of the family home in the child's new environment.
3. legal policy regarding allocation from the family home.

REFERENCES

Brady, S. (1980). Transitional Objects: Idealization of a Phenomena. *Psychoanalytic Quarterly, 40*; 561–595.

Bowlby, J. (1969). *Attachment and loss*, Vol I, London: Hogarth Press, p. 309–13.

Bowlby, J. (1961). Process of Mourning. *The International Journal of Psychoanalysis*, Vol XLII, Parts 4–7.

Busch, F. (1974). Dimensions of the first transitional object. *Psychoanalytic Study of the Child, 29*; 215–29.

Busch and McKnight, (1973). Parental Attitudes and the Development of Primary Transitional Objects. *Child Psychiatry and Human Development, 4*; 12–20.

Coppolillo, M. (1976). The transitional phenomena revisited. *Journal of American Academy of Child Psychiatry, 15*; 36–48.

DiLeo, Joseph (1973). *Diagnostic Aids*. Brunner/Mazel, NY.

Eissar, R.S. (1969). Object Constancy and Mental Representations. *The Psychoanalytic Study of the Child*, Vol 24, p. 9–47.

Gaddini, R., Gaddini, E. (1981). Transitional objects and the process of individuation. *Journal of American Academy of Child Psychiatry, 9*; 131–139.

Garrison, W. (1982). Attachment to a special object at the age of three years. Behaviour and Temperament Characteristics, *Child Psychiatry and Human Development, 12*(3).

Hetherington, E.M., Cox, M. (1978). The aftermath of divorce. In Stevens, J and Matthews, M., eds.: *Mother Child/Father Child Relationship*, Washington D.C., National Association for the Education of Young Children.

Hetherington, E., Cox, M. (1986). Prolonged Social Interaction in Children Following Divorce. *Journal of Social Issues*, in press.

Hong, Michael (1978). The Transitional Phenomena. *Psychoanalytic Study of the Child, 3*; 47–49.

Hong, Michael, K. (1976). Infant Attachment to Inanimate Objects. *Journal of Child Psychiatry, 15*; 49–61.

Isaacs-Elmhurst, Susan (1980). Transitional Objects in Transition. *International Journal of Psychoanalysis*, Vol 61.

Lichtenburg, Joseph (1979). Factors in the Development of the Sense of the Object. *Journal of the American Psychoanalytic Association*, Vol. 27.

Litt, Carole (1981). Children's Attachment to Transitional Objects. *American Journal of Orthopsychiatry, 51*(1).

Passman, R., Halmen, J. (1979). A developmental survey of young children's attachment to inanimate objects. *Journal of Genetic Psychology, 134*; 165–78.

Passman, R.H. (1977). Providing attachment objects to facilitate learning and reduce stress: effects of mothers and security blankets. *Developmental Psychology, 13*, 25–28.

Passman, R.H., (1976). Arousal reducing properties of attachment objects: testing the functional limits of the security blanket relative to the mother. *Developmental Psychology, 12*, 468–69.

Piaget, Jean (1965) *The Child's Conception of the World*. New Jersey, Littlefield, Adams and Co.

Piaget, Jean (1963). *The Origins of Intelligence in Children*. New York, W.W. Norton and Co.

Singer, J.L. (1977). Television, imaginative play and cognitive development: some problems and possibilities. Paper presented at *American Psychological Association Meeting*, San Francisco.

Thiveatt, R.W., (1980). Divorce; crises intervention guided by attachment theory. *American Journal of Psychotherapy, 34*(2).

Wallerstein, J. (1980). The Impact of Divorce on Children. *Psychiatric Clinics of North America*, Vol. 3, No. 3.

Wallerstein, J.S., Kelly, J.B. (1976). The effects of parental divorce: Experiences of child in latency. *American Journal of Orthopsychiatry, 46*, 256–269.

Wallerstein, J.S., Kelly, J. (1975). The effects of parental divorce: experiences of the preschool child. *American Academy of Child Psychiatry, 14*, 600–161.

Winnicott, D. (1953). Transitional objects and transitional phenomena, *International Journal of Psychoanalysis, 34* (part 2), 89–97.

Depression in Children from Single-Parent Families

Debra K. Huntley
Randy E. Phelps
Lynn P. Rehm

ABSTRACT. The study examined depression in 53 eldest children between six and ten years old who were living in mother-headed one-parent families. None of the children were involved in counseling or psychological treatment at the time of the study. Child report scores on the Children's Depression Inventory (CDI) were regressed on three variables, gender of the children, a self-report measure of the mother's depression, and the amount of time since the parents' separation. Analyses revealed that only gender of the child was a significant predictor of CDI scores, with boys reporting significantly greater depressive symptomatology. Contrary to expectation, neither time since separation nor depression in the mother added significantly to the prediction. Mother's ratings of the child on DSM-III criteria for depression were also regressed on the same three factors, revealing that only the mother's depression score was a significant predictor of her perceptions of the child's depressive symptoms. Results are discussed in terms of current models of the psychological effects of divorce on children.

In the U.S. today over 12 million families with children are headed by a single parent; over 83 percent of these parents are women (U.S. Census, 1980). Depression has often been cited as being evident in children experiencing the loss of a parent through

---

Debra K. Huntley, MA, is Doctoral Candidate, Department of Psychology, University of Houston—University Park, Houston, TX 77004.

Randy E. Phelps, PhD, is Assistant Professor, University of Texas Department of Psychiatry and Behavioral Sciences, Mental Sciences Institute, 1300 Moursund, Houston, TX 77030.

Lynn P. Rehm, PhD, is Professor, Department of Psychology, University of Houston—University Park, Houston, TX 77004.

This paper was presented at the annual meeting of the Texas Association of Marriage and Family Therapy, San Antonio, January, 1985. The research was supported in part by NIMH grant 37977 to the second author.

divorce (Child, 1980; Hetherington, 1979; Rickard, 1982; Wallerstein & Kelly, 1980). In fact, Caplan and Douglas (1969) indicate that loss of parents as a result of marital disharmony results in a higher incidence of depressive disorder than loss through death.

One of the most common early responses of the child to divorce is depression (Child, 1980; Hetherington, 1979). Furthermore, the first two years following the parent's separation appear to be the most difficult for the child, with problems adjusting to the loss of a parent greater during these two years than at any other time (Hetherington, Cox, & Cox, 1978). In contrast, however, Wallerstein and Kelly (1980) suggest that early affective responses to the divorce may extend over a much greater period of time. In their five-year follow-up of children of divorce, children were equally as likely to evidence the same affect and emotion as they did at the time of the separation.

Another factor related to depression in the child is gender. Harrington and Hassan (1958) and Kaslow, Rehm, and Siegel (1984) found that latency-aged girls appear to be more likely to evidence depression than boys. More recently, Lefkowitz and Tesiny (1985) reported that the prevalence rates for child depression were equal for both sexes in the general population. For children of divorce, however, studies indicate that the negative effects due to the separation of the parents are more severe for boys than for girls (Hetherington, 1979; Moreland, Schwebel, Fine, & Vess, 1982). The implication is that boys in these families may evidence more depressive symptomatology than girls.

There is also substantial evidence from the literature that children of depressed parents are themselves depressed (Cooper, 1977; Frommer, 1968; Kaslow, 1983; Poznanski & Zrull, 1970; Welner, Welner, McCrary, & Leonard, 1977). It has been suggested that depression interferes with the parent's ability to best meet the needs of the child, which results in subsequent psychopathology in the child in the form of depression or its equivalents (Philips, 1979). Rutter (1966), however, was unable to show a specific link between depression in the parent and depression in the child.

The present study examined the relative impact of each of these three variables, time since separation, gender of the child, and mother's depression on the child's depression using multiple regression procedures. Because of the controversy apparent in the literature on the difficulties associated with the description and measurement of childhood depression (Cytryn & McKnew, 1972; Deuber, 1982; Huntley, 1985) it was important to obtain multiple measures of the child's depression. This study utilized a child self-report measure, the

Children's Depression Inventory (CDI; Kovacs & Beck, 1977), and a conceptually-derived, mother-report measure based on the DSM III criteria for depression.

METHODS

Subjects

The sample consisted of 53 children, 29 boys and 24 girls between the ages of six and ten, and their mothers. The average age of the children was 7.80 years. These children were the eldest child in the family and the mothers were separated or divorced at the time of participation. The average length of time since the parent's separation was 52.6 months. In addition, the mother was the only adult in the home. Average income for these families was $1614 per month and the average education for the mother was 13.9 years.

Exclusion criteria for the children included the following: (1) no previous diagnosis of minimal brain dysfunction, mental retardation, or autism, (2) no reported incidence of physical or sexual abuse, (3) no previous diagnosis of psychosis, and (4) the child was not currently seeing a therapist, counselor, or minister for any type of psychological or behavioral problem.

Procedures

Subjects were recruited by notices in the newspapers, flyers, radio and television announcements, and talks given at community facilities. Interested subjects phoned in for further information, and if they met the criteria they were sent a packet including a consent form and study measures to fill out and return.

On return of these data, subjects were scheduled for an interaction task in the laboratory setting, which is not relevant to the present study. After completing the interaction, the child filled out the Children's Depression Inventory with the assistance of the examiner.

Instruments

A. Completed by the Child

Children's Depression Inventory (CDI; Kovacs & Beck, 1977). The CDI, a self-report inventory of 27 depressive items, was utilized to assess the child's self-report of his or her level of depression. The higher the total score, which ranges from 0 to 54, the more symptomatic the child was by his or her self-report. The CDI has acceptable levels of reliability and validity.

B. Completed by the Mother

Symptom Checklist (SCL-90; Derogatis, Lipman, & Covi, 1973). The SCL-90 is a self-report symptom inventory of 90 items with established validity and reliability which assesses various types of psychopathology. Each item can be rated on a 5-point scale of distress ranging from "not at all" to "extremely." The depression subscale of this measure was used to assess depression in the mother.

DSM-III Criteria for Major Depression.

This derived measure consisted of the nine symptoms listed in the DSM-III as criteria for major depression. Mothers were asked to indicate which of the nine items described the recent behavior of the child. Scores on the depression symptoms could range from 0 to 9.

RESULTS

Means, standard deviations, and bivariate correlations between all variables are displayed in Table 1. Note the lack of significance between the child's self report (CDI) and the mother's report of depression symptoms in the child. Due to this lack of correspondence, each variable was analyzed as a separate independent variable in subsequent analyses.

Separate multiple regression analyses was used to examine the relative impact of the predictor variables in the CDI and on the depression symptoms. In the first analysis, the CDI score was regressed on gender, the mother's SCL-90 depression subscale, and time (in months) since the separation or divorce. Variables were entered into the equation as listed in a fixed order.

Referring to Table 2, it is apparent that with all three variables in the equation, slightly more than 11% of the variance in CDI scores was accounted for, though the F-value of 2.054 for all three variables in was not significant. Of the three variables, only gender accounted for a significant proportion of the variance ($F = 5.371$; $p < .025$). Comparison of the mean CDI scores for both sexes revealed that boys scored significantly higher on this measure (boys: $M = 9.59$, $SD = 6.61$; girls: $M = 5.83$, $SD = 3.76$; $t = 2.32$, $p < .05$).

Table 1

Correlation Matrix, Means, and Standard Deviations
For All Variables

Measure	2	3	4	5	$\underline{M}$	$\underline{SD}$
1. CDI	.129	$-.309^{*}$	.106	.103	7.89	5.78
2. DSM III		.024	.146	$.582^{**}$	1.48	1.44
3. Gender			-.039	-.015	.43	.50
4. Time				.130	53.00	32.33
5. SCL-90 Depr.					1.26	.80

$^{*}p < .05$
$^{**}p < .001$

Table 2

Regression Analysis for CDI Measure

Predictor Variables	$\underline{R}^2$	$\underline{R}^2$ change	$\underline{F}$	$\underline{p}$
Gender	.095	.095	5.371	.025
SCL-90 Depr.	.105	.010	2.931	.063
Time	.112	.007	2.054	.119

In the second analysis, the mother's report of the child's depression on the DSM III measure was regressed on gender, mother's depression, and time, also in that order. Results are displayed in Table 3. The overall equation was highly significant ($F = 8.861$, $p < .0001$), accounting for almost 35% of the variance in the DSM III measure. However, inspection of Table 3

Table 3

Regression Analysis For DSM III Depression Symptoms

Predictor Variables	R^2	R^2 change	F	p
Gender	.001	.001	.031	.861
SCL-90 Depr.	.341	.340	13.168	.000
Time	.347	.006	8.861	.000

reveals that the mother's depression score on the SCL-90 alone accounted for 34% of the variance, with gender and time making only a negligible contribution.

DISCUSSION

In this study boys reported more depression than girls. This appears to be in contrast to recent data regarding prevalence rates of depression in children from the general population. Lefkowitz and Tesiny (1985), for example, found no sex differences in the prevalence of depression in a large sample of latency-aged children, suggesting that prior to puberty sex is not yet a risk factor for depression. Although this finding may hold for the general population, the current data suggest that boys who have lost a father to divorce may be at higher risk for depression than girls. This is consistent with other reports that boys are more likely to experience greater negative effects overall than girls following divorce (Hetherington, 1979).

In examining the mother's report of depression in the child, the only variable to account for a significant proportion of the variance was her own level of depression. If the mother was depressed, she tended to report her child as depressed. This finding is also consistent with those of other investigators who have shown that maternal depression significantly impacts the mother's perception of child maladjustment (Forehand, Wells, McMahon, Griest, & Rogers, 1982).

The amount of time elapsed since the parental breakup was unrelated to either the child's self-report of depressive symptoms or the mother's ratings. It may be that this finding is an artifact of characteristics of the present sample, in that the mean length of time since the separation was over four years. However, supplementary analyses comparing the depression measures for children whose parents had been separated for over two years with those whose parents had been separated less than two years revealed no significant differences. Nor were the depression scores distributed in a curvilinear fashion, as suggested by reports that adjustment difficulties peak at about one year following the breakup, and then become less severe over time (Hetherington, 1979). Instead, it appears that the passage of time itself may be a less important predictor of the adjustment of the child, as has been argued by Wallerstein and Kelly (1980), than other factors such as the mother's adjustment, the child's social network (Huntley & Phelps, 1985), patterns of parent-child interaction (Phelps & Slater, 1985) and the child's gender.

Interestingly, the correlation between the child's report of his or her own depression and the mother's report of depression in the child was not significant. Similar findings have been reported by Kazdin, French, and Unis (1983) for children on an inpatient unit, by Schultz, Rehm, and Siegel (1985), and by Kaslow, Rehm, Pollak, and Siegel (1985). They found that measures of depression completed by the children tended not to correlate with the same or related measures completed by the parents. While the lack of correspondence between child and parent ratings may bring into question the validity of the measures, it may also be that the different ratings reflect reliable and valid differences between the parent's and child's perception in identifying and reporting the child's depressive symptoms. Future research could address this question by incorporating additional sources of data such as teacher, peer, and interviewer reports.

REFERENCES

Caplan, M. & Douglas, V. (1969). Incidence of parental loss in children with depressive mood. *Journal of Child Psychology and Psychiatry, 10*, 225–232.

Child, A. (1980). Depression in children: Reasons and risks. *Pediatric Nursing*, July-August, 9–13.

Cooper, S. (1977). The children of psychiatric patients: Clinical findings. *British Journal of Psychiatry, 131*, 514–522.

Cytryn, L., & McKnew, D. (1972). Proposed classification of childhood depression. *American Journal of Psychiatry, 129*, 149–155.

Derogatis, L., Lipman, R., & Covi, L. (1973). The SCL-90: An outpatient psychiatric rating scale. *Psychopharmacology Bulletin, 9*, 13–28.

Deuber, C. (1982). Depression in the school-aged child: Implications for primary care. *Nurse Practitioner*, September, 26–30.

Frommer, E. (1968). Depressive illness in children. *British Journal of Psychiatry, Special Publications No. 2*, 117–136.

Forehand, R., Wells, K.C., McMahon, R.J., Griest, D., & Rogers, T. (1982). Maternal perception of maladjustment in clinic-referred children: An extension of earlier research. *Journal of Behavioral Assessment, 4*, 145–151.

Harrington, M. & Hassan, J. (1958). *British Journal of Medical Psychology, 31*, 43.

Hetherington, E.M. (1979). Divorce: A child's perspective. *American Psychologist, 34*, 851–858.

Hetherington, E., Cox, M. & Cox, R. (1978). The aftermath of divorce. In J.H. Stevens and M. Mathews (Eds.), *Mother-Child, Father-Child Relations*, Washington, D.C.: National Association for the Education of Young Children.

Huntley, D.K. (1985). *Depression in children from single-parent families and its correlates*. Unpublished master's thesis, University of Houston.

Huntley, D.K. & Phelps, R.E. (1985, April). *Depression and social contacts of children from one-parent families*. Paper presented at the meeting of the Southwestern Psychological Association, Austin, Texas.

Kaslow, N. (1983). *Depression in children and their parents*. Unpublished doctoral dissertation, University of Houston.

Kaslow, N., Rehm, L., & Seigel, A. (1984). Social-cognitive and cognitive correlates of depression in children. *Journal of Abnormal Child Psychology, 12*, 605–620.

Kaslow, N., Rehm, L., Pollak, S., & Siegel, A. (1985). *Attributional style and self-control behavior in depressed and nondepressed children and their parents*. Paper submitted for publication.

Kazdin, A.E., French, N.H., & Unis, A.S. (1983). Child, mother, and father evaluations of depression in psychiatric inpatient children. *Journal of Abnormal Child Psychology, 11*, 167–180.

Kovacs, M. & Beck, A.T. (1977). An empirical-clinical approach toward a definition of childhood depression. In J.G. Schulterbrandt and A. Raskin (Eds.), *Depression in childhood: Diagnosis, treatment, and conceptual models*, New York: Raven Press.

Lefkowitz, M.M., & Tesiny, E.P. (1985). Depression in children: Prevalence and correlates. *Journal of Consulting and Clinical Psychology, 53*, 647–656.

Phelps, R.E. & Slater, M.A. (1985). Sequential interactions that discriminate high- and low-problem single mother-son dyads. *Journal of Consulting and Clinical Psychology, 53*, 684–692.

Philips, I. (1979). Childhood depression: Interpersonal interactions and depressive phenomena. *American Journal of Psychiatry, 136*, 511–515.

Poznanski, E. & Zrull, J. (1970). Childhood depression. *Archives of General Psychiatry, 23*, 8–15.

Rickard, K., Forehand, R., Atkeson, B., & Lopez, C. (1982). An examination of the relationship of marital satisfaction and divorce with parent-child interactions. *Journal of Clinical Psychology, 11*(1), 61–65.

Rutter, M. (1966). *Children of sick parents*. Oxford University Press: Oxford.

Schultz, H., Rehm, L., & Seigel, A. (1985). *The assessment of depression in children and mothers*. Paper submitted for publication.

U.S. Bureau of the Census. (1980). Census of population: General, social, and economic characteristics. Washington, D.C., PC(1)-C1.

Wallerstein, J., & Kelly, J. (1980). *Surviving the breakup: How children actually cope with divorce*. New York: Basic Books.

Welner, Z., Welner, A., McCrary, D., & Leonard, M. (1977). Psychopathology in children of inpatients with depression: A controlled study. *Journal of Nervous Mental Disorders, 164*, 408–413.

Adolescents' Attitudes Toward Suicide: Does Knowledge That the Parents Are Divorced Make a Difference?

Jeffie A. Gibson
Lillian M. Range
Howard N. Anderson

ABSTRACT. Families of suicidal youths are viewed as more psychologically disturbed than families of youths who die from other causes, and experience other comparatively negative reactions as well. Likewise, divorced families also are viewed more negatively than intact families. To see whether a combination of suicide plus divorce led adolescents have particularly negative views, 120 high school students read one of four versions of a newspaper article about a teen's death. The teen was described as having lived either with both parents (I) or with his divorced mother (D), and as having died either from a rare disease (VI) or by suicide (S). As compared to VI teens and their parents, D teens and their parents were seen as more psychologically disturbed; and S parents were seen as more (a) to blame, (b) sad and depressed, (c) ashamed, and (d) in need of professional psychological help. As compared to I teens and their parents, D teens and their parents were seen as more psychologically disturbed, and, in the case of fathers, more unlikeable. Surprisingly, these students expected to have less trouble expressing sympathy to divorced parents than to intact parents. However, a combination of divorce and suicide did not exacerbate the negative perceptions and anticipated reactions of these high school students.

The authors are on the faculty, Department of Psychology, University of Southern Mississippi.

Portions of this manuscript were presented at the annual meeting of the Southeastern Psychological Association, Atlanta, March, 1985. Address reprint requests to Lillian M. Range, PhD, Department of Psychology, Southern Station Box 5025, Hattiesburg, MS 39406-5025.

Adolescents affected by divorce may demonstrate a wide range of psychological reactions, including anger, fear, depression, guilt (Hetherington, 1979; Sorsky, 1977; Wallerstein & Kelly, 1976), behavior disorders, neurotic conflicts, and psychotic breakdowns (Sorosky, 1977). Some investigations have even found that divorced families are particularly common among suicidal youths and suicide attempters (Dorpat, Jackson, & Ripley, 1969; Hawton, 1982).

An additional source of stress frequently encountered by children from divorced homes is that many people expect them to have problems whether they actually do or not. Santrock & Tracy (1978) vividly illustrated this phenomenon by asking teachers to rate boys from two-parent (intact) homes or divorced homes. Teachers rated boys from divorced homes as unhappier, more emotionally maladjusted, and less able to cope with stress, than boys from intact homes.

This result raises the question of whether or not negative views of youths and their divorced parents would occur in another negative situation, such as a youth's suicide. If so, divorced parents of a suicidal adolescent would experience particularly negative reactions from community members as compared to nondivorced parents of a suicidal adolescent, or to parents of a child who died of a rare disease. Such were the hypotheses of the present study.

METHOD

Subjects

Participants were a representative sample of 120 high school juniors and seniors (47 boys, 73 girls) from an urban public high school in the southeast. They ranged in age from 14 to 19, with an average age of 16.8 years.

Materials

Variations of brief newspaper articles (adapted from Calhoun, Selby, & Faulstich, 1980) were prepared which described a 16-year-old boy who died. In one version, the death was a suicide (S); and, the boy had lived with both parents (I). In a second version, the death was again a suicide (S); but, the parents were divorced (D), and the boy lived with the mother. In a third version, the death was from a rare disease (R); and the boy had lived with both parents (I). In the fourth version, the death was from a rare disease (R), and the parents were divorced (D), with the boy living with the mother.

Except for type of death and marital status of the parents, the articles were identical.

A short questionnaire (also adapted from Calhoun et al., 1980) accompanied each of the newspaper articles. It contained some demographic questions and 19 Likert-type items which were designed to assess the respondents' attitudes toward the adolescent who died and the bereaved family.

Procedure

Students were asked during study hall if they would be willing to participate in research dealing with people's reactions to serious childhood incidents. If so, they were given consent forms to take to their parents. Those who returned signed forms (88.4% of all parental forms were returned) were then given their own consent forms. Those who returned both consent forms (81.6%) read one of the four randomly assigned variations of the newspaper articles, and then anonymously responded to the questionnaire.

RESULTS

Chi square analyses indicated no significant differences between groups in age or gender. A two way multivariate analysis of variance yielded a significant effect for type of death, $F(19,98) = 7.50$, $p < .001$, and for marital status of parents, $F(19,98) = 2.81$, $p < .001$, but no significant multivariate interaction.

A priori t tests for the type of death predictions indicated significant effects on eight of the 19 variables. First, S youths were seen as more psychologically disturbed (''moderately disturbed'') than R youths (''essentially normal and well adjusted''), $t(116) = 10.23$, $p < .001$. Second, S fathers were rated as more psychologically disturbed (''slightly'') than R fathers (''essentially normal and well-adjusted''), $t(116) = 2.10$, $p < .05$. Third and fourth, blame was greater for S mothers (''slight'') and fathers (''moderate'') than for R mothers (''essentially blameless'') and fathers (''slight''), $t(116) = 2.51, p < .01$ and $t(116) = 2.35, p < .05$, respectively. Fifth and sixth, sadness and depression were expected to last longer for S mothers (''four to six years'') and fathers (''three years'') than for R mothers (''two years'') and fathers (''two years''), $t(116) = 4.34$, $p < .01$ and $t(116) = 4.04$, $p < .001$, respectively. Seventh, S families were thought to have more reason to be ashamed (''a little reason'') than R families (''absolutely no reason''), $t(116) = 3.10, p < .001$. Eighth, S families were thought to need help from a mental health professional (''slightly agree'') more so than R families (''neutral''), $t(116) = 2.44, p < .01$.

A priori t tests for the marital status predictions indicated significant effects on four of the 19 variables. First, D youths were seen as more psychologically disturbed (''moderately'') than I youths (''mildly''), $t(116) = 2.14, p <$ 05. Second and third, D fathers and mothers were seen as more psychologically disturbed (''mildly'') than I fathers and mothers (''essentially normal and well adjusted''), $t(116) = 4.34, p < .001$, and $t(116) = 3.55, p < .001$, respectively. Fourth, D fathers were expected to be liked less (''neutral'') than I fathers (''slightly positive''), $t(116) = 2.52, p < .01$.

Further univariate analyses indicated that, contrary to predictions, respondents expected to have more difficulty (''moderate difficulty'') in expressing sympathy to I families than to D families (''neutral''), $F(1,116) = 8.18, p < .001$. No additional univariate analyses, and no univariate interactions, reached statistical significance.

DISCUSSION

The comparatively negative attitudes of these high school students toward suicide victims and the bereaved family are similar to the attitudes of adults (Calhoun et al., 1980; Range, Bright, & Ginn, 1985; Rudestam & Imbroll, 1983) and older adolescents (Gordon, et al., in press). Likewise, the comparatively negative attitudes toward divorced parents and their children are similar to adult attitudes (Santrock & Tracy, 1978).

It was interesting that although divorce resulted in the parents as well as the youth being seen as psychologically disturbed, it did not affect other aspects of how the parents and family were perceived (except likeability of the father, which was also negatively affected). Divorced parents were expected to be sad and depressed, blamed, etc., following the death of their child the same as parents who were together. Thus, being divorced affected how psychologically healthy parents were perceived to be, but not how they were expected to react to their child's death.

The one exception to the above generalization was the surprising finding that these high school students thought that expressing sympathy to the bereaved family would be easier if the parents were divorced than if they were together. Perhaps the divorced parent was seen as having no spouse to lean on for emotional support, and therefore more in need of emotional support and sympathy than parents who lived together and presumably had each other.

Also surprising was that the neither the multivariate interaction nor any of the univariate interactions were significant. Thus, a combination of divorce and suicide did not exacerbate the negative perceptions and anticipated reactions of these high school students.

An implication of these results is that intervention with bereaved parents must deal not only with their grief, but also with whatever negative impact may result from others knowing either the nature of the death or the fact that they are divorced. Of course, when interpreting results of attitudinal research, one must be aware that the correspondence between self-reports of reactions to hypothetical victims and bereaved families may not correspond to actual behavior toward those who are personally known. Nevertheless, studies such as this one may assist mental health professionals to become more aware of existing attitudes so that they might take steps to prepare grieving parents to deal with the reactions of others in the community.

REFERENCES

Calhoun, L. G., Selby, J. W., & Faulstich, M. E. (1980). *Journal of Consulting and Clinical Psychology, 48*, 535–536.

Dorpat, T. L., Jackson, J. D., & Ripley, H. H. (1969). Broken homes and attempted and completed suicides. *Archives of General Psychiatry, 12*, 213.

Gordon, R. S., Range, L. M., & Edwards, R. P. (in press). Generational differences in reactions to adolescent suicide. *Journal of Community Psychology.*

Hawton, K. (1982). Annotation: Attempted suicide in children and adolescents. *Journal of Child Psychology & Psychiatry & Allied Disciplines, 23*, 497–503.

Hetherington, E. M. (1979). Divorce: A child's perspective. *American Psychologist, 34*, 851–858.

Range, L. M., Bright, P. L., & Ginn, P. D. (1985). Public reactions to parents of a child suicide: Effects of child's age and method used. *Journal of Community Psychology, 13*, 288–294.

Rudestam, K. E. & Imbroll, D. (1983). Societal reactions to a child's death by suicide. *Journal of Consulting and Clinical Psychology, 51*, 461–462.

Santrock, J. W. & Tracy, R. L. (1978). Effects of children's family structure status on the development of stereotypes by teachers. *Journal of Educational Psychology, 70*, 754–757.

Sorosky, A. D. (1977). The psychological effects of divorce on adolescents. *Adolescence, 12*, 123–136.

Wallerstein, J. S. & Kelly, J. B. (1976). The effects of parental divorce: Experiences of the child in later latency. *American Journal of Orthopsychiatry, 46*, 256–269.

Young Adult Children of Divorced Parents: Depression and the Perception of Loss

Rebecca L. Drill

ABSTRACT. Results of a questionnaire study of the long-term effects of divorce in young adults of divorced parents indicate that depression is related to the young adult's perception of the parents, rather than to the divorce itself. Specifically, when the non-custodial parent is perceived as "lost," the young adult is more depressed. When a divorce occurs, the perception of the non-custodial father has been shown to change in a negative direction, while the perception of the mother (whether custodial or non-custodial) remains relatively stable. These results have implications for intervention.

The number of children affected by divorce is on the rise. In 1974, little more than a decade ago, over one million children under the age of eighteen had been touched by the divorce of their parents (Wallerstein & Kelly, 1976a). This number now stands at over three million (Statistical Abstract of the United States: 1981), and the upward trend seems to be continuing. The fact that so many children are affected by the divorce experience has called attention to the need for continuing research in the area, and many researchers have responded to the call. Their findings, however, are complex and varied, and often raise more questions than they answer.

Most researchers seem to agree that depression is a prominent and frequent effect of parental divorce on children (Gardner, 1976; McDermott, 1970, 1968; Wallerstein & Kelly, 1980, 1977, 1976a,

---

Rebecca L. Drill, PhD, is Clinical Fellow at Harvard University. Correspondence should be sent to the author at: 12 Commonwealth Avenue, Boston, MA 02116.

This paper is a revised version of a doctoral dissertation submitted to the faculty of the Gordon F. Derner Institute of Advanced Psychological Studies at Adelphi University. This paper received a Meritorious Award from the New York State Psychological Association in the graduate level of the clinical division in the 1985 competition.

1976b). However, a variety of reasons has been hypothesized for this depressive reaction. Most investigators postulated that depression is related to some type of loss—of the family unit, of the parental unit, of the departed father (Hetherington, Cox, & Cox, 1976; Jacobson, 1978; McDermott, 1968; Prinz, Bella, & Oppenheimer, 1983; Wallerstein & Kelly, 1980, 1976a, 1976b).

Others have concluded that the remaining parent can compensate for the loss (Pett, 1982; Rosenthal, 1979). The author believes that such a loss, specifically of the non-custodial parent (not necessarily always the father), cannot be resolved entirely by the presence of the other parent, for that child has formed a primary bond with both parents, and the breaking of that bond with one of them can only be felt as a tragic loss. Bowlby (1980) and Caplan and Douglas (1969) have described parental loss as a causal factor of depression in children (Bowlby, 1980) and in adults (Caplan & Douglas, 1969).

Although in reality the departed parent may not be "lost," as in the event of death, the loss may be felt just as strongly (although perhaps in a different manner) in the case of a divorce. For this reason, what is most important is the child's *perception* of the loss of the non-custodial parent. It is this perception that is crucial to the child's post-divorce functioning. While the non-custodial parent is not necessarily the father, it should be recognized that, indeed, the father *is* usually the non-custodial and absent parent; most children from divorced families live with the mother. However, cases where the mother is the non-custodial parent were included in this study, as parental gender is not believed to be the critical factor in the parent-child relationship (Rosen, 1979; Santrock & Warshak, 1979).

While these initial ideas may not be novel to this field, this author proposes to take them one step further. The research conducted on the long-term effects of divorce is inconsistent and complex (Chess, Thomas, Korn, Mittleman, & Cohen, 1983; Grossman, Shea, & Adams, 1980; Hainline & Feig, 1978; Kulka & Weingarten, 1979; Kurdek, Blisk, & Siesky, 1981; Landis, 1960; Mendelsohn, 1982; Rutter, 1971; Stolberg, Camplair, Currier, & Wells, 1983; Wallerstein & Kelly, 1980), and points to many factors suggested to be responsible for different outcomes. Some studies have concluded that effects persist for years after the divorce (Landis, 1960; Wallerstein & Kelly, 1980), while others have concluded that they do not (Grossman et al., 1980; Hainline & Feig, 1978; Kulka & Weingarten, 1979; Kurdek et al., 1981).

It seems that in some children the effects last, while in others they do not. Yet, some factors must be critical in this *differential* long-term outcome. Thus, it is hypothesized that the persistence of the young adult's perception of the non-custodial parent will affect the long-term consequences of the divorce on the young adult. If the child continues to perceive the non-custodial parent as a loss, the child will be depressed in young adulthood. Conversely, if the child does not continue to perceive the non-custodial parent as a loss, the immediate depressive reaction will have abated before young adulthood.

The divorce per se is not seen as the essential factor in determining depression; rather, the perception of parental loss is associated with the depression. Therefore, a child from an intact home who perceives one parent as "lost" should also be depressed like the child from the divorced home. However, it is hypothesized that the divorce situation is more likely to be associated with the perception of parental loss, since the parent is often physically, as well as emotionally, gone from the child's life. Therefore, children from divorced homes are more likely to perceive a parent as lost.

While "loss" itself is not measurable quantitatively, a similar idea, the "attitude" an individual holds toward the lost object, can be measured. The research reviewed suggests this attitude is primarily negative in the case of divorce, apparently because the parent is no longer involved in the child's life and because there has been an increase in the emotional distance between the departed parent and the child (Landis, 1960; McDermott, 1968; Wallerstein & Kelly, 1976b).

The author studied depression in young adults by examining their current perception of both parents, specifically focusing on the non-custodial parent. The subjects were college students, 18 to 23 years of age, from both divorced and intact families. A non-clinical population was used in an attempt to eliminate outside factors relating to depression and the perception of loss which are more likely to be found in a clinical population irrespective of parental marital status.

The analyses not only attempt to ascertain if a relationship does indeed exist between the perception of the non-custodial parent and current depression, but also examines whether this perception transcends the background variables of divorced vs. intact families, as well as demographic and attitudinal variables. The implications of a significant relationship may indicate that the perception of parental loss, rather than the divorce experience per se, is the primary factor in persisting depression among the children of divorce.

HYPOTHESES

1. Children of divorced parents will be more depressed than children of non-divorced parents.
2. Children of divorced parents will show a less favorable attitude toward the non-custodial parent than toward the custodial parent.
3. When the father is the non-custodial parent, children of divorced parents will rate their fathers less favorably than will children of non-divorced parents.
4. When the mother is the custodial parent, children of divorced parents will rate their mothers more favorably than will children of non-divorced parents.
5. Children of divorced parents will show greater discrepancy between their attitudes toward their parents than will children of non-divorced parents.
6. Children who show a greater discrepancy between their attitudes toward each parent, regardless of family status, will be more depressed than children who rate both parents equally.
7. Children who rate their parents discrepantly and are from divorced families will be more depressed than all other children.

METHOD

Subjects

The subjects in this study were young adults between the ages of 18 and 23, who were students in classes at five colleges in the New York/New Jersey Metropolitan area. The classes chosen included a range of introductory courses so that students with different interests would be represented within the study.

Subjects from intact homes served as the control group. Those from broken homes due to death were excluded, as were those either outside of the specified age range or who had omitted more than a small number of questionnaire items. Exclusive of these subjects (N = 238), the initial data collection yielded 104 students from divorced families and 276 from intact families. Because the proportion of students from divorced and non-divorced backgrounds at each college differed, the number of subjects included in the study from each college was adjusted to approximate the highest percentage of "divorce" subjects found at any one school. The highest ratio found was five "divorce" subjects to every eight "non-divorce" subjects. Because of rounding, a 5:8 ratio could only be approximated. Using this proportion, the adjustment was made for each college sample using the Random Sampling Table. The final subject pool consisted for 104 students from divorced families and 172 from non-divorced families.

Procedure

A packet of questionnaires was distributed to the undergraduate students participating in the study. Students were asked not to complete the questionnaires if they had already done so in another class. It was also stressed that they should fully answer each of the questions. The packet included the following: (1) a consent form, (2) the Attitudes Toward Parents Scale (Form F for fathers and Form M for mothers), (3) the Multiple Affect Adjective Check List—General Form, and (4) a demographic and attitudinal questionnaire. The questionnaires took approximately 30 minutes to complete. Participating students were offered the option of receiving the results of this study.

Measures

Attitude Toward Parents Scale

Itkin (1952) developed the "Attitudes Toward Parents Scale" as part of a battery of scales to measure attitudes related to the family. This scale consists of two forms: Form F for measuring attitudes toward the father and Form M for measuring attitudes toward the mother. The forms are identical except for the use of "father" or "mother" respectively. The Attitudes Toward Parents Scale consists of 35 items—11 true/false/uncertain questions, 8 multiple choice questions, and 16 personality traits which are self-rated on a five point scale. Each of the possible alternatives is given a numerical value, which is not presented to the subjects. The attitude score is calculated by totalling the values of each item endorsed. The possible score on each form ranges from 46 to 164, with a high score indicating a more favorable attitude toward parents.

Split-half reliabilities were .92 (corrected to .96) for form F and .85 (corrected to .92) for form M. Internal consistency analyses showed item validity to be strong. External validity was tested by correlating attitude scores with self-rating scores where low self-ratings and high attitude scores indicated favorable attitudes toward parents. Scores on Form F correlated −.70 with self-ratings and those on Form M correlated −.80 with self-ratings. Itkin and outside reviewers of the scale have recommended its use in research concerned with attitudes toward parents.

Multiple Affect Adjective Check List

Zuckerman and Lubin's (1965) Multiple Affect Adjective Check List (MAACL) is an extension of their original Affect Adjective Check List. The MAACL consists of two forms—a "General" form and a "Today" form—which are designed to provide stable trait and brief state measures, respectively, of the following three affects: anxiety, depression, and hostility. Since this study assessed long-lasting depression, only the General form was employed. Therefore, only it will be reviewed.

The MAACL is a self-administered test containing 132 adjectives which are listed in alphabetical order. Forty items are used to assess depression, twenty-eight to assess hostility, and twenty-one to assess anxiety. The remaining forty-three are buffer items which are not scored. Some endorsed items indicate the presence of a specific affect ("+" items) while others indicate that affect's absence ("0" items). Subjects are asked to mark an "X" in the box next to those words which describe how they *generally* feel. Each of the three affects (anxiety, depression, hostility) is individually scored on its own scale. The total score for each scale is calculated by adding the number of "+" items which are endorsed with the number of "0" items which are *not* endorsed.

The General form was expected to show high internal (split-half or item inter-correlation) reliability and high test-retest reliability. It is difficult to fully assess the reliability of the MAACL's General form since reliability research has only focused on the Anxiety scale of the General form (r = .68), and on the Today form of the full MAACL (as reported in Zuckerman and Lubin, 1965). However, according to E.I. Megargee (Buros, 1972), the addendum to the scale manual reports coefficients of .70, .65, and .54 for the Anxiety, Depression, and Hostility scales, respectively.

A similar problem exists regarding validity research of the MAACL General form—the majority of the research has concentrated upon either the Anxiety Scale only or upon the MAACL Today form. Once again, however, Megargee presented some additional information. He stated that the Anxiety and Depression scales (form not specified) generally correlate with clinical ratings of these dimensions, but the covergent validity of the Hostility scale is less adequate. Overall, the Anxiety scale has been given the most attention, and reviewers seem to consider it to be the most valid measure of the three. Zuckerman and Lubin (1965) stated that the General Anxiety scale ''may be used to obtain a quick estimate of the general level of anxiety (anxiety as a trait)'' (p.22). In regard to the Depression and Hostility scales, however, the writers note that the scales ''have not yet been assessed for this purpose but it is possible that they could serve as substitutes for longer questionnaires'' (p. 22). The authors and outside reviewers suggest that the MAACL has been used effectively and successfully in a variety of research projects.

RESULTS

Hypothesis 1 states that children of divorced parents will be more depressed than the children of non-divorced parents. Depression was measured by the Multiple Affect Adjective Check List (Zuckerman and Lubin, 1965). A multiple regression was used to test this hypothesis. The hypothesis was not supported, $F(4,150) = .02$. The data are presented in Table 1.

Hypothesis 2 states that children of divorced parents will show a less favorable attitude toward the non-custodial parent than toward the custodial parent. Attitude toward parent was measured by the Attitudes Toward Parent Scale (Itkin, 1952). A t-test was used to support this hypothesis. This hypothesis was supported, $t(63) = 5.09$, $p < .01$, 2-tailed.

When only those subjects living with their fathers were examined (N = 11), no significant variation between their attitudes toward each parent was found, $t(10) = .21$. Similarly, when only those subjects who alternate between each of their parents' homes were

TABLE 1
Multiple Regression

Dependent Variable: Depression
Predictor Variable: Parents' Marital Status

Variable	Multiple R	B	Standard BETA	Error B	F
Length of time in Therapy	0.24553	-4.285755	-0.22448	1.54512	7.694**
Number of Siblings	0.24849	-0.1426103	-0.03045	0.37332	0.146
Parents' Income	0.26205	0.7139613E-05	0.08342	0.00001	1.032
Parents' Marital Status	0.26228	-0.1501769	-0.01132	1.06808	0.020

(Constant) 18.87127

*p<.05
**p<.01

examined (N = 5), there was no significant variation found between attitudes toward each parent, t (4) = 2.19.

Hypothesis 3 states that when the father is the non-custodial parent, children of divorced parents will rate their fathers less favorably than will children of non-divorced parents. Attitude toward father was measured by Form F of the Attitudes Toward Parents scale (Itkin, 1952). Using a multiple regression to test this hypothesis, the hypothesis was supported, $F(4,129) = 6.317$, $p < .01$. The data are presented in Table 2.

Hypothesis 4 states that when the mother is the custodial parent, children of divorced parents will rate their mothers more favorably than will children of non-divorced parents. Attitude toward mother was measured by the M Form of the Attitudes Toward Parents Scale (Itkin, 1952). A multiple regression was used to test this hypothesis. This hypothesis was not supported, $F(4,129) = .091$. The data appear in Table 3.

While this hypothesis was not supported, other findings were significant. A Pearson Correlation was done which suggested a significant relationship between status and attitude toward father, r = .3577, $p < .01$. Children of divorce rated their fathers less

TABLE 2
Multiple Regression

Dependent Variable: Attitude Toward Father
Predictor Variable: Parents' Marital Status

Variable	Multiple R	B	Standard BETA	Error B	F
Length of time in Therapy	0.23893	16.33271	0.23478	5.71251	8.175**
Number of Siblings	0.23955	0.4750949	0.02872	1.35882	0.122
Parents' Income	0.30681	0.8602339E-04	0.21219	0.00003	6.634**
Parents' Marital Status	0.36935	10.43612	0.20682	4.15222	6.317**

(Constant) 68.58498

*p<.05
**p<.01

TABLE 3
Multiple Regression

Dependent Variable: Attitude Toward Mother
Predictor Variable: Parents' Marital Status

Variable	Multiple R	B	Standard BETA	Error B	F
Length of time in Therapy	0.14785	8.459442	0.14351	5.11273	2.738*
Number of Siblings	0.16946	1.231569	0.08786	1.21615	1.026
Parents' Income	0.18943	0.3001689E-04	0.08738	0.00003	1.008
Parents' Marital Status	0.19121	1.121074	0.02622	3.71626	0.091

(Constant) 113.2227

*p<.05
**p<.01

favorably than did children of non-divorce. Status and attitude toward mother were not significantly related, r = .0782.

T-tests were also performed comparing the attitudes toward each parent in all non-divorce group subjects with those divorce group subjects who live with their mothers. Divorce group subjects who live with their fathers (N = 11) and those who alternate living with each parent (N = 5) were excluded because of their small number. Children of divorce living with their mothers rated their fathers significantly less favorably than did children of non-divorced parents, $t(81.74) = -4.76$, $p < .01$, 2-tailed, while there was no significant difference between the two groups when rating their mothers, $t(86.46) = -1.02$.

Hypothesis 5 states that children of divorced parents will show a greater discrepancy between their attitudes toward each of their parents than will children of non-divorced parents. Attitude discrepancy is the absolute value of attitude toward mother subtracted from attitude toward father. A multiple regression was performed. This hypothesis was supported, $F(4,150) = 7.650$, $p < .01$. The data are presented in Table 4.

Hypothesis 6 states that children, regardless of parents' marital

TABLE 4
Multiple Regression

Dependent Variable: Discrepancy Between Attitudes Toward Parents
Predictor Variable: Parents' Marital Status

Variable	Multiple R	B	BETA	Standard Error B	F
Length of time in Therapy	0.06977	-4.443341	-0.07850	4.58269	0.940
Number of Siblings	0.07282	-0.6922788E-01	-0.00499	1.10722	0.004
Parents' Income	0.14308	-0.4203730E-04	-0.16567	0.00002	4.066**
Parents' Marital Status	0.26078	-8.761979	-0.22287	3.16783	7.650**

(Constant) 46.94012

*p<.05
**p<.01

status, who show a greater discrepancy between their attitudes toward each parent will be more depressed than children who rate both parents equally. A multiple regression was done which yielded significant results, and thus, the hypothesis was supported, $F(4,150) = 3.537$, $p < .01$. The data are presented in Table 5. A Pearson Correlation showed that a larger discrepancy was significantly associated with a greater degree of depression, $r = .1687$, $p < .01$.

Pearson Correlations followed which showed that a less favorable attitude toward father was significantly correlated with greater depression, $r = -.2707$, $p < .01$, and a less favorable attitude toward mother was also correlated with greater depression, $r = -.2815$, $p < .01$.

Hypothesis 7 states that children who rate their parents unequally and are from divorced families will be more depressed than all other children. ''Unequally'' was defined by those attitude ratings which were one or more standard deviations discrepant. Using a multiple regression, this hypothesis was not supported, $F(4,150) = 1.145$. The data appear in Table 6.

A Pearson Correlation was then conducted using the same data, again yielding insignificant results, $r = -.0794$. Although this correlation is not statistically significant, the findings are in the expected direction—children from divorced families who rated their parents unequally tend to be more depressed.

The same multiple regression used to test Hypothesis 7 (data presented in Table 6) revealed that the most significant contribution to the intensity of depression is the length of time in therapy, $F(4,150) = 7.759$, $p < .01$. A Pearson Correlation revealed that a longer time in therapy was associated with a lesser degree of depression, $r = .2267$, $p < .01$.

Post-Hoc Analyses

An analysis of variance and covariance with repeated measures was performed for between and within groups of children of divorce and non-divorce regarding their attitude toward mother and toward father, $F(1,274) = 12.93$, $p < .01$. The differences were significant. HSD procedures followed. The data are presented in Tables 7A and 7B.

TABLE 5
Multiple Regression

Dependent Variable: Depression
Predictor Variable: Discrepancy Between Attitudes Toward Parents

Variable	Multiple R	B	BETA	Standard Error B	F
Length of time in Therapy	0.24553	-4.031135	-0.21114	1.52940	6.947**
Number of Siblings	0.24849	-0.1451393	-0.03099	0.36837	0.155
Parents' Income	0.26205	0.8911896E-05	0.10412	0.00001	1.670
Attitude Toward Parents Discrepancy	0.30021	0.4992012E-01	0.14800	0.02654	3.537**

(Constant) 16.97751

*p<.05
**p<.01

TABLE 6
Multiple Regression

Dependent Variable: Depression
Predictor Variable: Parents' Marital Status and Discrepancy Between Attitudes Toward Parents

Variable	Multiple R	B	Standard BETA	Error B	F
Length of time in Therapy	0.24553	-4.275194	-0.22393	1.53478	7.759**
Number of Siblings	0.24849	-0.1510716	-0.03226	0.37142	0.165
Parents' Income	0.26205	0.7442760E-05	0.08696	0.00001	1.164
Parents' Marital Status and Attitude Toward Parents Discrepancy	0.27518	-1.779780	-0.08404	1.66360	1.145

(Constant) 21.98726

*p<.05
**p<.01

TABLE 7
Attitude Towards Parents
Post-hoc Analyses

Table 7A

Analysis of Variance and Covariance with Repeated Measures

Dependent Variables: attitude toward father, attitude toward mother

Source	Sum of Squares	Degrees of Freedom	Mean Square	F	Two-tailed Probability
Mean	8408603.78918	1	8408603.78918	15218.02	0.0000
Status	18764.30369	1	18764.30369	33.96	0.0000
Error	151396.68907	274	552.54266		
Emotion	30674.24777	1	30674.24777	78.08	0.0000
ES	5081.35646	1	5081.35646	12.93	0.0004*
ERROR	107638.13629	274	392.83991		

*p<.01

Table 7B

Significant Differences of Within- and Between-Group Means Using Tukey-HSD Procedure

Attitude Towards Parents of Divorce and Non-divorce Groups

	M_1	M_2	M_3	M_4
Divorce Group Attitude Toward Father M_1 = 110. 50962	---	21.644**	18.293**	---
Divorce Group Attitude Toward Mother M_2 = 132. 15385		---	---	5.77
Non-divorce Group Attitude Toward Father M_3 = 128. 80233			---	9.12209**
Non-divorce Group Attitude Toward Mother M_4 = 137. 92442				---

**significant for HSD, 2-tailed

Within group analysis showed that both children of divorce and children of non-divorce rate their mothers more favorably than they rate their fathers. Between group analysis showed that this discrepancy in rating, while significant for both groups, was greater for the divorce group. A substantial main effect was found for parental gender, with the divorce group rating their fathers significantly less favorably than did the non-divorce group. The divorce group rated their mothers less favorably than did the non-divorce group, but this trend was not statistically significant.

DISCUSSION

Major Findings

Hypothesis 1 states that children of divorced parents will be more depressed than children of non-divorced parents. This hypothesis was not supported, but the finding is consistent with the author's proposed view that it is not the divorce itself which is related to depression. Rather, there must be some other factor associated with long-term characterological depression in the children of divorce.

The critical variable proposed was the perception of the loss of the non-custodial parent. In the case of divorce, a parent is not "lost" to the same extent as in the reality of death. However, in some instances, that parent may be perceived by the child as totally uninvolved in the child's life and, therefore, experienced as "lost." It is this perception which may be directly related to the long-term post-divorce adjustment of the child.

Since divorce is a situation which is conducive to viewing one parent as lost, it was expected that the departed ("non-custodial") parent might be viewed in a less favorable light. Other researchers have studied the non-custodial parent's role in the divorce process and have concluded that the non-custodial parent-child relationship is important to the child's adjustment (Hetherington et al., 1976; Jacobson, 1978; Landis, 1960; Prinz et al., 1983; Wallerstein & Kelly, 1977). While most projects have singled out the father as the non-custodial parent, studies indicate that the gender of the custodial parent is not significant (Rosen, 1979; Santrock & Warshak,

1979). This study included cases where the mother as well as the father was the non-custodial parent, as the parent's sex was not expected to be the determining factor in the child-parent relationship.

Therefore, Hypothesis 2 states that children of divorced parents will show a less favorable attitude toward the non-custodial parent than they do toward the custodial parent. This hypothesis was supported, and the overwhelming majority of cases were ones in which the mother was the custodial parent. In the cases where the father remained involved (11 father-custody and 5 joint-custody cases), he was *not* rated significantly more negatively than the mother. Interestingly, when the mother was the non-custodial parent, she also was not rated less favorably. This indicates that the attitude towards the divorced father tends to be more negative when he is the non-custodial parent, while the attitude towards the divorced mother remains stable regardless of the status of custody.

Hypotheses 3 and 4 were designed in order to compare the attitudinal discrepancy toward parents between children of divorce and those of non-divorce. Hypothesis 3 states that when the father is the non-custodial parent, children of divorced parents will rate their fathers less favorably than children of non-divorced parents. This hypothesis was supported. Hypothesis 4 states that when the mother is the custodial parent (i.e., the father is the non-custodial parent), children of divorced parents will rate their mothers more favorably than will children of non-divorced parents. This hypothesis was not supported.

Post-hoc analyses followed in order to clarify the issue of parental sex vis-à-vis custody. The results were consistent with the findings discussed thus far. Children of divorce seem to have a more negative perception of their fathers than do children of intact marriages. However, there were no significant differences between the perceptions of children of divorce and those of non-divorce regarding their mothers.

Hypothesis 5 states that children of divorce will show a greater discrepancy between their attitudes toward their parents than will children of non-divorce. This hypothesis was supported. A stringent post-hoc test revealed that children of both divorced and non-divorced parents rated their mothers more favorably than they rated their fathers. While this discrepancy was significant for both groups, it was greater in the case of divorce, as these children rated their fathers significantly less favorably than did children of non-divorce.

Hypothesis 6 states that children who show a greater discrepancy between their attitudes toward each parent, regardless of their parents' marital status, will be more depressed than children who rate both parents equally. This hypothesis was supported. In fact, a larger discrepancy was significantly associated with greater depression. A less favorable attitude toward the father was also significantly associated with greater depression, as was a less favorable attitude toward the mother.

The findings from this study highlight the importance of the continued involvement of the father after a divorce, and therefore have implications for the father-child relationship both during and after the divorce process. These findings also support other studies which have found significant correlations between children's positive adjustments and their positive evaluations of their parents (Kurdek & Siesky, 1980). Furthermore, this evidence underscores the importance of a child's "perception," rather than the actual "reality" of the situation.

Hypothesis 7 states that children who rate their parents unequally and are from divorced families will be more depressed than other children. This hypothesis was not supported, although the trend was in the expected direction. The negative results are not surprising, however, since it has been shown that the divorce itself is not the crucial factor in depression. Thus, the inclusion of parents' marital status in this hypothesis diluted the predictive value of the discrepant parental ratings.

Interestingly, when both discrepant parental ratings and parents' marital status were examined simultaneously, the only variable found to be significantly related to the degree of depression was the length of time in psychotherapy. As the time in therapy increased, the degree of depression lessened. This finding highlights the use of psychotherapy as an effective means of helping depressed children after a parental separation or divorce.

Suggestions for Future Research

A major finding of this study was the importance of the non-custodial parent's continued relationship with the child following a divorce. Further research might more fully investigate the effects of joint-custody. Another finding was that there was a negative change in the attitude towards the father, but not towards the mother, which occurred as the result of a divorce. Further research might explore the conditions leading to and causing such a change. A third finding involved the child's tendency to perceive the non-custodial parents as "lost" following divorce. Further research might compare the depression resulting from this perception to the situation of a child who has lost a parent through death.

Implications for Intervention

The results of this study have strong implications for constructive ways of dealing with the divorce situation. The study reveals that long-term effects may occur following a divorce, even though it is not the divorce itself that is the villain. Perception of loss appears to play a major role in the long-term consequence of depression. Regardless of the "reality" of the loss of a parent, a child's perception of loss seems to be the operative factor. Psychotherapy is apparently an effective method of dealing with the depression and sense of loss which may affect a child after a divorce.

Because divorce is a process, not an isolated event, the effects of the divorce may be cumulative and early intervention would therefore be beneficial. The continued involvement of the non-custodial parent in the child's life appears crucial in preventing an intense sense of loss in the child, while psychotherapy may function as both a preventive and remedial measure. The importance of the relationship with the non-custodial parent may also have implications for the legal issues of custodial arrangements and visitation. The results of this study indicate that arrangements where both parents are equally involved with the child are optimal. When this type of arrangement is not possible, the child's continued relationship with the non-custodial parent remains essential.

REFERENCES

Bowlby, J. (1980). *Loss: Vol. III. Attachment and loss*. New York: Basic Books.

Buros, O.K. (Ed.). (1972). *The Seventh Mental Measurements Yearbook* (Vol. 1., pp. 269–274). Highland Park, NJ: The Gryphon Press.

Caplan, M.G., & Douglas, V.I. (1969). Incidence of parental loss in children with depressed mood. *Journal of Child Psychology and Psychiatry, 10*, 225–232.

Chess, S., Thomas, A., Korn, S., Mittleman, N.M., & Cohen, J. (1983). Early parental attitudes, divorce and separation, and young adult outcome: Findings of a longitudinal study. *Journal of the American Academy of Child Psychiatry, 22*, 47–51.

Gardner, R. A. (1976). *Psychotherapy with children of divorce*. New York: Jason Aronson.

Grossman, S. M., Shea, J. A., & Adams, G.R. (1980). Effects of parental divorce during early childhood on ego development and identity formation of college students. *Journal of Divorce, 3*, 263–272.

Hainline, L., & Feig, E. (1978). The correlates of childhood father absence in college-aged women. *Child Development, 49*, 37–42.

Hetherington, E. M., Cox, M., & Cox, R. (1976). Divorced fathers. *The Family Coordinator, 25*, 417–428.

Itkin, W. (1952). Some relationships between intra-family attitudes and pre-parental attitudes toward children. *The Journal of Genetic Psychology, 80*, 221–252.

Jacobson, D.S. (1978). The impact of marital separation/divorce on children: I. Parent-child separation and child adjustment. *Journal of Divorce, 1*, 341–360.

Kulka, R. A., & Weingarten, H. (1979). The long-term effects of parental divorce in childhood on adult adjustment. *Journal of Social Issues, 35*, 50–78.

Kurdek, L. A., Blisk, D., & Siesky, A. E., Jr. (1981). Correlates of children's long-term adjustment to their parents' divorce. *Developmental Psychology, 17*, 565–579.

Kurdek, L. A., & Siesky, A. E., Jr. (1980). Effects of divorce on children: The relationship between parent and child perspectives. *Journal of Divorce, 4*, 85–99.

Landis, J. T. (1960). The trauma of children when parents divorce. *Marriage and Family Living, 22*, 7–13.

McDermott, J. F. (1970). Divorce and its psychiatric sequelae in children. *Archives of General Psychiatry, 23*, 421–427.

McDermott, J. F. (1968). Parental divorce in early childhood. *American Journal of Psychiatry, 124*, 1424–1432.

Mendelsohn, R. (1982). *Divorce, depression, perceived maternal depression and autonomy*. Unpublished doctoral dissertation, Adelphi University.

Pett, M. G. 1982. Correlates of children's social adjustment following divorce. *Journal of Divorce, 5*, 25–39.

Prinz, R. J., Bella, B. S., & Oppenheimer, K. C. (1983, August). *Children of separating parents: They are not all alike*. Paper presented at the 91st Annual Convention of the American Psychological Association, Anaheim, CA.

Rosen, R. 1979. Some crucial issues concerning children of divorce. *Journal of Divorce, 3*, 19–25.

Rosenthal. P. A. (1979). Sudden disappearance of one parent with separation and divorce: The grief and treatment of preschool children. *Journal of Divorce, 3*, 43–54.

Rutter, M. (1971). Parent-child separation: Psychological effects on the children. *Journal of Child Psychology and Psychiatry, 12*, 233–260.

Santrock, J. W., & Warshak, R. A. (1979). Father custody and social development in boys and girls. *Journal of Social Issues, 35*, 112–125.

Statistical Abstract of the United States: 1981. 102 ed. U.S. Dept. of Commerce: Bureau of the Census.

Stolberg, A. L., Camplair, C., Currier, K., & Wells, M. J. (1983). *Individual, familial, and environmental predictors of children's post-divorce adjustment and maladjustment*. Unpublished manuscript, Virginia Commonwealth University, Richmond, VA.

Wallerstein, J. S. & Kelly, J. B. (1980). *Surviving the breakup: How children and parents cope with divorce*. New York: Basic Books.

Wallerstein, J. S. & Kelly, J. B. (1977). Brief interventions with children in divorcing families. *American Journal of Orthopsychiatry, 47*, 23–39.

Wallerstein, J. S. & Kelly, J. B. (1976a). The effects of parental divorce: Experience of the child in later latency. *American Journal of Orthopsychiatry, 46*, 256–269.
Wallerstein, J. S. & Kelly, J. B. (1976b). The effects of parental divorce: Experiences of the child in early latency. *American Journal of Orthopsychiatry, 46*, 20–32.
Zuckerman, M., & Lubin, B. (1965). *Manual for the Multiple Affect Adjective Check List.* San Diego: EdITS.

FAMILY REORGANIZATION

Recoupling: Development and Establishment of the Spousal Subsystem in Remarriage

Judith A. Kvanli
Glen Jennings

ABSTRACT. This paper discusses the results of an exploratory study that investigated the development and establishment of the spousal subsystem in remarriage following divorce. The strengths of nonclinical couples were also investigated. Data were gathered by analyzing videotaped in-depth interviews of 10 remarried couples, all of whom were in their second or subsequent marriage following divorce. The mean length of time of the remarriages was 7.8 years. The developmental tasks of the remarriage process including first marriage, divorce, and courting, were recounted by 20 remarried husbands and wives. The findings indicated the individuals experienced increasing differentiation and supportive relationships with their families of origin during the divorce/remarriage cycle. The stages of courting and early remarriage emerged as themes that described developmental sequences of experiences that were reflective of individual and couple tasks during each of the periods. As the tasks of the early period of remarriage were completed, each spousal subsystem gradually experienced a recoupling process, that is,

Judith A. Kvanli, MS, is Marriage and Family Therapist, 3201 Broken Bow, Denton, TX 76201.

Glen Jennings, EdD, is Professor, Department of Family and Consumer Studies, Texas Women's University, Denton, TX 76201.

perceived the occurrence of an emotional bonding. The relationship patterns that evolved were representative of the period of stabilized established remarriage. The strengths of the remarried couples in the study emerged in the following themes: couple focusing, positive attitudes towards change, mutual acceptance of differences between the spouses, self-awareness, marital conflicts viewed as learning experiences, and minimal illusions of remarriage. Implications for counselors, family-life educators, and therapists who work with remarried couples or couples who are considering remarriage following divorce are suggested.

The liberalization of the Divorce Act in 1968 has enabled many couples to legalize their divorce and to remarry. Over three fourths of the divorced persons remarry within three to five years of their divorce (Norton & Glick, 1976). The number of divorces granted in the United States in 1978 was close to half the number of marriages (National Center for Health Statistics, 1980). According to Glick's (1983) review of the 1980 Current Population Survey, five years after entry into marriage formerly married persons have a 50% greater probability of divorce; at 10 years, the risk of divorce among remarriers is 20% greater; by 25 years, it is less than 10% greater. As a result of Duberman's (1975) study of the future of marriage, it is estimated that more people will be living in a second marriage than in a first marriage by the end of the century.

Messinger (1982) reports that socialization in the nuclear family provides an inadequate model for the variety of remarriage structures. A conceptual model is required that can reflect the various structures of remarriage. The results of these studies indicate that there is a large population living in family systems for which they have not been prepared.

While there have been many studies in recent years that focus on remarriage from the perspective of the entire stepfamily system, there is a dearth of research that has investigated stabilized remarried spousal subsystems following divorce. Marital happiness in remarriage was researched by Albrecht (1979); Glenn and Weaver (1977); and White (1979). Garfield (1980) researched the decision to remarry and presented a profile for readiness for remarriage and outlined the process by which divorced people decide to remarry. The importance of the couple bond in remarriage is addressed by Beal (1980); Messinger (1976); and Whiteside (1982).

Furstenberg (1979) states that family sociologists are disinclined to acknowledge the complexity of the remarried spousal system. They continue to treat divorce and remarriage as departures from an accepted marriage practice rather than as regularities in a changing system of kinship. There is little information about the problems that people experience as they move through the transitions from one marriage to the next.

Remarriage is emerging as a common form of marriage (Goetting, 1982). At the present time, remarriages represent 32% of all marriages in the United States (Price-Bonham & Balswick, 1980). Furstenberg (1979) introduced the concept "normative schedule" to explain the demographic processes that become relatively constant over time. That is, marriage, divorce and subsequent remarriage have become part of the life course.

According to McGoldrick and Carter (1980), the complexity of the remarriage process requires adding an additional phase to the family life cycle. As the first marriage signifies the joining of two families, subsequent marriages involve the interweaving of three, four, or more families. For stabilization to occur and the forward developmental thrust to continue following divorce, those who are involved in the process experience a separate developmental stage. This requires that specific developmental tasks be accomplished. As Kleinman, Rosenberg, and Whiteside (1979) report, the formation of a solid marital relationship, despite the past failures of the remarried couple, is one of the most challenging tasks of the remarried couple. This period of reorganization presents special tasks for the remarried couple.

Wald (1981) addressed three key concepts that are central to the psychosocial development of the remarried couple: the life cycle stage of the couple, the developmental tasks required for that stage, and the existing emotional bonds of the couple. The process of bonding begins at birth and normally takes place in one's family of origin. A process of bonding occurs again in the marital relationship.

Bonding in remarriage is tedious because intimacy is difficult to achieve. The couple that does not bond is often pulled apart by their old attachments and cannot function as a viable subsystem. The couple cannot perform as a couple unit and adequately lead the family (Goldner, 1982). Previous relationship difficulties often lead to a need for comfort in the new relationship. This pseudomutuality, a desperately happy facade (Goldstein, 1974), often prevents the resolution of difficulties in the new relationship.

When the couple remarries, there is a social expectation that the remarried couple will remain married throughout old age and form emotional bonds and attachments similar to the emotional bonds in the first marriage (Wald, 1981, p.124). This expectation is often frustrated because of the greater complexities for the remarried couple such as the existence of former spouses and the lack of acceptance from kinship networks.

This study was grounded by family systems theory (Bowen, 1976). The six interlocking concepts of the theory include triangles, the nuclear family emotional process, the family projection process, the differentiation of self, the multigenerational transmission process, emotional cutoffs, and sibling position (Bowen, 1974). This theoretical foundation guided the interpretations of the authors.

In summary, the study explored the development and establishment of the spousal subsystem in remarriage following divorce. Of special interest was the influence of the family of origin and former spouse on the spousal subsystem, the individual and couple tasks of the divorce/remarriage cycle, and the perceived strengths of each remarried couple. The authors systematically coded and analyzed the perceptions and experiences of the couples at the completion of videotaped in-depth interviews.

METHOD

The major questions of this exploratory study were: what factors influenced the development and establishment of the nonclinical spousal subsystem in remarriage following divorce and what were the perceived strengths of the remarried couples? These questions were answered through the process of videotaped in-depth interviews and the clinical impressions of the authors.

Sample

The sample consisted of 10 remarried couples who volunteered to participate in the study. All of the spouses had been divorced and had been in their current remarriage for a minimum of four years, had not received marital counseling during their remarriage, were not currently experiencing marital problems or problems with a child and were in good physical health. Subjects were accepted for the study when both partners agreed to participate, each stated that they felt content in the remarriage, and when both partners fulfilled the eligibility requirement of scoring at or above the normative sample mean of 114 on the Dyadic Adjustment Scale (Spanier, 1976). This self-report instrument measures dyadic cohesion, marital adjustment, dyadic consensus, marital satisfaction, and overt affection. The subjects were all white and, based on educational levels, represented a middle class population. The average length of time between marriages of the sample was 2.0 years and the average length of time in the previous marriage was 8.9 years. The mean length of time in the current marriage was 7.8 years. Each of the subjects was in a second marriage with the exception of one who was in a third marriage. The mean age of the subjects was 39.4 years. The average number of children between the spouses was 2.3 and all individuals were Protestant, with the exception of two who were Catholic.

Procedures

The data used to answer the research questions were taken from systematic coding and analysis of the data from videotaped in-depth interviews and the clinical impressions of the authors. The interviews took place in the participants' homes. The format of the interviews was semi-structured. The participants received the Personal Authority in the Family System Questionnaire (Williamson, Bray, and Malone, 1983). This self-report instrument assesses important relationships in the three generational family system. The subjects' scores on the following subscales of the *PAFS* were assessed in this study: spousal fusion, spousal intimacy, intergenerational intimidation, intergenerational intimacy, intergenerational fusion, intergenerational triangulation, and personal authority. The subjects' scores on seven of the subscales provided support for the findings of this study (Table 1).

RESULTS

Differentiation from the Family of Origin and Former Spouse

The informants recounted positive relationships with their families of origin during the time of the divorce/remarriage cycle. The themes that emerged were indicative of parental friendships, parental support, and low levels of parental involvement in the lives of the

Table 1

PAFS Subscales

Spouse	SPINT	SPFUS	ININT	INFUS	INTRI	INTIM	PERAUT
W1	55	90	123	36	45	134	62
H1	55	84	118	38	33	123	58
W2	54	60	90	28	50	113	40
H2	52	48	85	31	22	110	37
W3	55	63	113	38	13	119	54
H3	55	63	78	31	13	136	42
W4	52	66	90	25	32	108	43
H4	55	60	112	35	34	125	56
W5	47	64	121	37	11	81	50
H5	47	68	104	34	32	82	46
W6	54	75	110	37	55	103	50
H6	46	67	103	36	25	112	36
W7	46	63	90	30	47	131	42
H7	48	63	87	32	28	127	46
W8	55	79	103	31	18	110	44
H8	53	76	106	34	18	138	52
W9	47	64	85	21	14	111	42
H9	46	70	88	36	27	92	57
W10	54	63	93	28	14	104	45
H10	54	63	100	35	36	110	54
Possible Range	11-55	20-100	25-125	8-40	11-55	29-145	18-63
Normative:							
Mean	45.2	64.6	93.6	29.5	27.0	98.6	42.1
St.Dev.	8.2	8.4	17.3	5.2	11.7	24.9	8.0
Sample Mean W:	51.9	68.7	101.8	31.1	29.9	111.4	47.8
H:	51.1	66.2	98.1	34.2	26.8	115.5	48.4
All:	51.5	67.4	100.0	32.6	28.4	113.4	48.1

Description of PAFS Subscales Used in the Study

SPINT: Spousal Intimacy Subscale
These items assess the degree of intimacy and satisfaction with their mate.
Higher scores indicate more intimacy.

SPFUS: Spousal Fusion/Individuation Subscale
These items measure the degree to which a person operates in a fused or individuated manner in relationship with the mate.
Higher scores indicate more individuation.

ININT: Intergenerational Intimacy Subscale
These items assess the degree of intimacy and satisfaction with parents.
Higher scores indicate more intimacy.

INFUS: Intergenerational Fusion/Individuation Subscale
These items measure the degree to which a person operates in a fused or individuated manner with parents.
Higher scores indicate more individuation.

INTRI: Intergenerational Triangulation Subscale
These items measure triangulation between a person and his/her parents.
Higher scores indicate less triangulation.

INTIM: Intergenerational Intimidation Subscale
These items measure the degree of personal intimidation experienced by an individual in relation to his/her parents.
Higher scores indicate less intimidation.

PERAUT: Personal Authority Subscale
These items reflect topics of conversation which require an intimate interaction with a parent, while maintaining an individuated stance.
Higher scores indicate more personal authority.

remarried couples. Of special interest was the increasing differentiation from the family of origin during the time of the divorce, courting, and remarriage period. These transitions had provided opportunities for these divorced individuals to perceive themselves as increasingly independent from their families of origin and to develop adult to adult relationships with their families of origin during these periods.

Relationships with former spouses were not significant issues for the respondents at the time of the study. For some, relationships with former spouses had been relevant factors in the earlier period of remarriage and issues during that period often focused on children and parenting responsibilities. Former spousal relationships were frequently utilized as baselines for assessing the current remarriage relationship. Dysfunctional behavior patterns from the first marriage were remembered as a sense of déjà vu.

Recoupling Issues

Trust

Building trust in remarriage was considered a challenge as well as a crucial determinant to the establishment of the spousal subsystem. The development of trust was a gradual process that evolved over a period of years. The losses experienced as a result of the previous marriage significantly influenced the individuals' ability to develop trust in the remarriage relationship.

Friendships

Many of the spouses in the study reported experiencing 'best friend' relationships with their current spouse. Satisfactions in the remarriage were derived from genuinely liking each other, not taking each other for granted, knowing what they wanted from a spouse in the current marriage, and being able to confide in each other.

Acceptance of Differences

The remarried spouses often expressed positive feelings regarding complimentary styles of communication, behavior patterns, and interests. Differences were viewed as being beneficial to the remarried relationship, opportunities for growth, and challenges for self-improvement.

Effects of Change

The influence of change was addressed by several of the respondents. The individuals viewed these changes as a result of three factors: life cycle changes, the process of maturation, and purposeful changes. Life cycle events, e.g., the birth of a child and children leaving the nest, were viewed as opportunities to learn new and more adaptable styles of relating to each other. Many of the spouses recounted having been aware of their own maturing process by feeling a sense of contentment, reevaluating priorities, and becoming more flexible in relationships.

Individual and Couple Tasks of Early Remarriage

Individual Tasks

The adjustment to remarriage involved giving up previous single images and lifestyles as well as unfinished business from the past. Several of the wives discussed the challenges of giving up careers after remarriage. This had been a decision based on a desire to prioritize the remarriage. Giving up old hurts and grievances was also a task for the individuals making the transition to remarriage.

Couple Tasks

The management of conflict was a common task of the early remarriage period. What couples fought over was not as important as how the conflicts were resolved. The interaction with children and former spouses was a common source of conflict in the early remarriage period.

As the couples adjusted and made the necessary individual and couple accommodations during the early period of remarriage, the emergence of bonding gradually appeared. The couples expressed feelings of closeness, contentment, and blending in the remarriage relationship.

Individual Tasks Required to Move from First Marriage to Remarriage

First Marriage

Perceptions of the former marriage were recounted by the informants and were reflective of self-understanding regarding their decision to marry the first time. Several individuals expressed awareness of inappropriate reasons for marrying previously. Decisions had been based on wanting to get away from home, having a need to be independent of their families, marrying the most available person, and marrying because of social or family pressures.

Divorce

Divorce was viewed as a learning experience and the discomfort of the process was recognized. Several individuals had experienced parental divorce as children and expressed disappointment in repeating the divorce process in their own lives. This transition had been an opportunity to evaluate themselves and accept some responsibility for the dissolution of the previous marriage. Many of the individuals recounted this period as having been a time of developing adult to adult relationships with their families of origin. This was indicative of the increasing differentiation of the individuals from their families of origin during this transition. For others, the divorce increased their awareness of new dimensions of themselves as well as what they wanted in a partner the second time around.

Singlehood

The period of singlehood was viewed as a time of freedom, having a good time, and doing things they had never done before. Other respondents viewed this time as a period to heal wounded egos and enhance self-images.

Courting

Courtship was experienced as a time of caution and self protection and several of the informants stated that they had needed time alone after the divorce. This realization came after they became involved in a relationship during their divorce process or shortly after the legal divorce. A brief courtship was experienced by one couple and they stated that they hoped others considering remarriage would not follow their lead. Others expressed the belief that they had met their current spouse at an appropriate time; they had learned to feel good about themselves and were aware that they were satisfied and content without a partner. When relationships evolved and commitments were made they were based on choice, not personal or financial necessity. Several of the couples had planned for the foreseeable challenges of remarriage. Frequently mentioned topics of discussion were children, in-laws, and individual psychological struggles.

Strengths of Remarried Couples

Commitment to the remarriage was a central theme of the remarried spouses. Many of the couples stated that their remarriage was sucessful because they 'worked' at it and each spouse was equally committed to making the relationship work. Being able to learn from mistakes and having flexible roles were recounted by several individuals as being significant factors in the development of the spousal relationship. Prioritizing the remarriage was recognized as a crucial factor by many of the couples.

Several of the couples spent time getting to know each other before remarriage. As a result, they believed they had viewed each other realistically before remarriage. Many expressed belief in the deception of the dating process and adhered to the idea that a small amount of tension in the relationship before remarriage was helpful. This allowed each individual to become aware of their potential mate's response to stress prior to remarriage.

The themes of the remarried spousal subsystem development and establishment are summarized in Table 2. The findings include the perceptions and experiences of husbands and wives.

CONCLUSIONS

The effect of the family of origin on the development and establishment of the spousal subsystem was a finding of the study. The increasing level of differentiation of the remarried spouses from their families of origin was indicated by several themes. The couples had developed friendships with their parents and there was a balance between togetherness and separateness. Perceived parental interference was acknowledged by some remarried individuals. A resolution of problems with the family of origin was actively pursued and the increasing differentiation of the spouses from their families of origin was apparent. Individual differentiation was evidenced in various contexts during the transitional periods from first marriage to remarriage. The individual scores on the following subscales of the Personal Authority in the Family System Question-

Table 2

Themes of the Spousal Subsystem Development in Remarriage
Perceptions and Experiences of Husbands and Wives

	H	W	Total
Current Remarriage			
Family of origin issues			
Parental friendships	5	6	11
Parental support	3	4	7
Recoupling Issues			
Trust	4	7	11
Spousal friendships	6	5	11
Acceptance of differences	8	7	15
Positive effects of change	8	5	13
Early Remarriage			
Individual issues			
Single image alteration	3	4	7
Careers	0	5	5
Priorities	5	2	7
Couple issues			
Conflict resolution	7	4	11
Conflict areas			
Children	2	3	5
Former spouses	3	0	3
Bonding	3	5	8
First Marriage, Divorce, Singlehood			
Marrying for wrong reason	5	3	8
Family support during divorce	6	7	13
Self-evaluation following divorce	7	7	14
Divorce as a learning experience	3	3	6
Singlehood as productive time period	6	4	10
Courtship			
Viewed as a cautious period	5	3	8
Planned for challenges of remarriage	6	4	10
Strengths of Remarried Couples			
Commitment and effort	5	4	9
Knowing partner before remarriage	3	8	11
Expectation of change	6	5	11
Minimal illusions	8	7	15
Flexible roles	4	6	10
N =	10	10	20

naire (Williamson, Bray, and Malone, 1983) support these findings: intergenerational intimacy, intergenerational fusion, intergenerational triangulation, intergenerational intimidation, and personal authority (Table 1).

If there had been parental disapproval during the divorce/remarriage cycle, this had been resolved prior to or during the development of the remarriage. For the most part, the couples viewed their relationships with their parents and parents-in-law favorably. There appeared to be a low level of fusion between the remarried spouses and their families of origin at the time of the study.

Involvement with former spouses was limited to parenting issues during the later period of remarriage. Relationships with former spouses were indicative of minimal fusion and gradual differentiation between these spouses had evolved following the legal divorce.

This study suggests that the development of trust was a prerequisite for the establishment of the spousal subsystem in remarriage. Trust building required a period of time and gradually evolved as an emotional bonding occurred between the spouses. This experience signified the completion of one of the couple tasks in the early remarriage period and was indicative of the movement into the established remarriage period.

Spousal friendships were important dimensions in established remarriage. These friendships were not representative of fused relationships, but well differentiated marital relationships. The couples moved in and out of the marital relationship and demonstrated a balance of separateness and togetherness. These findings are supported by the quantitative data from the spousal intimacy and spousal fusion subscales on the *PAFS*.

Acceptance of differences was a significant finding of the couples in the study. This is further evidence for the similar level of differentiation of the spouses (Bowen, 1978). Lack of sameness was welcomed and viewed as a significant factor in the functioning of the relationship. Many of the spouses were able to maintain "I" positions regarding differences, including conflict.

Change was recognized as a naturally occurring phenomenon and the remarried couples recalled many occasions when they had acknowledged the expectation of change, not only individually but in the couple context. On an individual level, change often occurred as the result of maturation, experience, or deliberate decision making (Bernard, 1973). In the context of the couple, changes frequently occurred as a result of the natural evolution of the life cycle and commitment to making the relationship work.

The transition from singlehood to remarriage was portrayed as a period of individual and couple adjustments. Giving up roles and careers as singles were important issues. The resolution of conflict in the period of early remarriage often involved each spouse's awareness and acknowledgment of their own dysfunctional patterns of relating in the previous marriage.

The satisfactions of the remarried couples centered around general feelings of contentment, a stage of blending for the remarried couples. Closeness between the remarried spouses was maintained as they experienced frequent individual changes and couple challenges throughout the transitions of the remarriage.

Some respondents viewed the marriage that ended in divorce as an opportunity to either leave home and develop independence or fulfill parental and/or social expectations. A high level of fusion with the family of origin was apparent during the experience of first marriage and divorce for many individuals.

Many individuals viewed the experience of divorce as a learning experience. The influence of parental divorce in the lives of some of the respondents left scars that maintained their sensitivity. Evidence of high levels of emotional fusion in the nuclear family had been their childhood experience. Several informants were committed to not replicating the divorce experience and stated their belief in the importance of self-evaluation following a divorce.

Many individuals stated that parental support was available following the separation from their former spouse, even though this transition required a period of readjustment for the extended families. The divorce adjustment period had provided opportunities for the individual's continued differentiation from their families of origin. The less differentiated individuals and their families experienced a longer and more stressful period of readjustment.

The post divorce period was a time for continued individual differentiation for some informants. It was a time for self evaluation, ego building, and emotional recovery.

Courtships often evolved into living together situations and the respondents stated that these arrangements provided "not always glamorous" day to day settings for developing their relationships. Courtship was a viewed as a period of caution by several couples and some planned for the challenges of remarriage.

The establishment of the remarried spousal subsystem was explained by some couples as a result of communication, commitment, and prioritizing the remarriage. Other couples placed an emphasis on the importance of knowing each other before remarriage and the willingness of each partner to modify and alter non-productive patterns of behavior remembered from the previous marriage.

This study provides implications for those professionals who work with remarried couples following divorce. Frequently these couples have become derailed in the developmental process of establishing the spousal subsystem in remarriage. The study also provides implications for those counselors and educators who provide guidance for those couples who are considering remarriage in the future.

The results of the study apply directly to 20 divorced/remarried spouses who are representative of a white, middle class population from the North Texas area. Other kinds of populations, such as those representing a more generalizable sample, may provide additional data that will enhance the current research. Finally, the evidence accumulated here clearly indicates that the development and establishment of the spousal subsystem in remarriage is an individual and couple process and recoupling must be considered as more than an event in the life cycle. Those spouses who shared their retrospective accounts of the process of remarriage, as well as their perceptions of the strengths of remarriage, have allowed the authors to code and analyze the data and scientifically report the findings of this study. The important task of future research will be to further investigate the development and establishment of the spousal subsystem in remarriage and consider this subsystem's functioning as part of a three generational process. Most importantly, the development and establishment of this subsystem must be considered an integral part of the process of stepfamily system formation.

REFERENCES

Albrecht, S. (1979). Correlates of marital happiness among the remarried. *Journal of Marriage and the Family, 41*, 857–867.

Beal, E. W. (1980). Separation, divorce and single-parent families. In E. A. Carter & M. McGoldrick (Eds.). *The family life cycle: A framework for family therapy*. New York: Gardner Press.

Bernard, J. (1973). *The future of marriage*. New York: Bantam Books.

Bowen, M. (1976). Theory in the practice of psychotherapy. In P. Guerin (Ed.), *Family therapy*, New York: Gardner Press.

Bowen, M. (1978). *Family therapy in clinical practice*. New York: Jason Aronson.

Duberman, L. (1975). *The reconstituted family: A study of remarried couples and their children*. Chicago: Nelson-Hall.

Furstenberg, F. F., Jr. (1979). *Recycling the family: Experiences in remarriage*. Philadelphia: Center for Research on the Acts of Man.

Garfield, R. (1980). The decision to remarry. *Journal of Divorce, 4,* 1–10.

Glenn, N. D. & Weaver, C. N. (1977). The marital happiness of remarried divorced persons. *Journal of Marriage and the Family, 39,* 331–337.

Glick, P. C. (1983). Prospective changes in marriage, divorce, and living arrangements. *Journal of Family Issues, 1,* 455–479.

Goetting, A. (1982). The six stations of remarriage: Developmental tasks of remarriage after divorce. *Family Relations, 31,* 213–222.

Goldner, V. (1982). Remarriage family: Structure, system, future. In J. C. Hansen & L. Messinger (Eds.), *Therapy with remarriage families*, Rockville, MD: Aspen.

Goldstein, H. S. (1974). Reconstituted families: The second marriage and its children. *Psychiatric Quarterly, 48,* 433–440.

Kleinman, J., Rosenberg, E., & Whiteside, M. (1979). Common developmental tasks in forming reconstituted families. *Journal of Marital and Family Therapy, 5,* 79–86.

McGoldrick, M., & Carter, E. (1980). Forming a remarried family. In E. Carter & M. McGoldrick (Eds.), *The family life cycle: A framework for family therapy*. New York: Gardner Press.

Messinger, L. (1976). Remarriage between divorced people with children from previous marriages: A proposal for preparation for remarriage. *Journal of Marriage and Family Counseling, 2,* 193–200.

Messinger, L. (1982). *Therapy with remarriage families*. Rockville, Maryland: Aspen System Publication.

National Center for Health Statistics (1980). Births, marriages, divorces, and deaths for 1979. Monthly Vital Statistics Report (Vol. 28), No. 12, Provisional Statistics. Hyattsville, Maryland: U.S. Department of Health, Education, and Welfare.

Norton, A. J., & Glick, P. C. (1976). Marital instability: Past, present and future. *Journal of Social Issues, 32,* 5–20.

Price-Bonham, S., & Balswick, J. O. (1980). The noninstitutions: Divorce, desertion, and remarriage. *Journal of Marriage and the Family, 42,* 959–972.

Spanier, G. B. (1976). Measuring dyadic adjustment: New scales for assessing the quality of marriage and similar dyads. *Journal of Marriage and the Family, 38,* 15–28.

Wald, E. (1981). *The remarried family: Challenge and promise*. New York: Family Service Association of America.

White, L. (1979). Sex differentials in the effects of remarriage on global happiness. *Journal of Marriage and the Family, 41,* 869–876.

Whiteside, M. F. (1982). Remarriage: A family developmental process. *Journal of Marital and Family Therapy, 8,* 59–68.

Williamson, D. S., Bray, J. H., & Malone, P. E. (1983). *Personal authority in the family system questionnaire*. Houston Family Institute.

Defining Post-Divorce Remarriage Families: A Typology Based on the Subjective Perceptions of Children

Penny Gross

ABSTRACT. The central question addressed in this study is membership in a post-divorce remarriage family, i.e., how are its boundaries to be defined. In sociology the remarriage family has been traditionally and inappropriately defined within the nuclear family paradigm.

An alternative manner of investigation is looking at how the participants themselves define their families. In this study sixty children in remarriage families were asked whom they considered to be members of their families.

A typology of four mutually exclusive and exhaustive types was developed based on children's subjective perceptions of parental family membership. Respondents were found in all four types: retention, substitution, reduction and augmentation. On an exploratory basis, variables were examined which might account for respondent's location in one of these four types.

The findings in this study have important implications for the definition of family after divorce and remarriage and call for a recognition of the importance of the children's perspective.

A major difficulty confronting those who wish to analyze remarriage families, is the lack of an adequate theoretical framework (Esses and Campbell, 1984). In family sociology generally, the nuclear or first marriage family is regarded as the prototype of normality, or the "gold standard" of family structure. Implicitly

---

Penny Gross, PhD, is Visiting Scholar at The Ontario Institute for Studies in Education, Department of Sociology, 6th Floor, 252 Bloor Street West, Toronto, Ontario, Canada M5S 1V6.

The author wishes to thank Margrit Eichler for her invaluable assistance.

and explicitly other family structures are compared to the nuclear family. This has led to a common approach in analyzing remarriage families called "deficit-comparison" (Ganong and Coleman, 1984), with the underlying assumption that any non-nuclear family has "problems" simply due to its structure.

An alternative way of looking at the lack of fit between the nuclear model and other types of families, is to question the supremacy of the model. Because of societal changes which have a direct impact on family structure, not *all* family forms fit into our existing model. The nuclear model was designed for a time when families were more structurally uniform; it has now been suggested that within the context of divorce and remarriage we must rethink our conceptualization of the family in sociological research (Bumpass, 1984).

The perspective taken in this study is to regard the nuclear model itself as lacking in flexibility. Its structure is rigid, unable to accommodate the "fluid" (Eichler, 1983) or "permeable" (Messinger et al., 1978) boundaries that now exist for many types of families. In this study, a way of looking at remarriage families is described, which moves beyond the superimposing of the nuclear family model.

RATIONALE

Although it is recognized by clinicians that nuclear families and remarriage families are very different (for example, see Sager et al., 1983), on a theoretical level remarriage families continue to be treated as recreated nuclear families. For example, in a Statistics Canada publication on divorce, remarriage is seen as "a greater commitment to living in a *workable* nuclear family. . ." (Statistics Canada, 1983, emphasis in the original). The sociological definition of remarriage family is also a replica of the nuclear model: "any remarriage which includes at least one child residing in the household of the remarriage spouses" (Price-Bonham and Balswick, 1980).

The remarriage family is different from the nuclear family and these differences prevent the remarriage family from fitting neatly into the nuclear model format. In a remarriage family, a divorced parent remarries and new of acquired kin, generally referred to as "stepkin," enter the scene. These stepkin do not readily fit into any existing models of kinship. Kinship analysts have referred to them as "quasi-kin" (Bohannan, 1971) and "relatives-in-law" (Schneider, 1980). As kin acquired after divorce and remarriage, they are a relatively new phenomenon, having increased substantially in number over the last three decades.

There is a second problem in trying to fit remarriage families following divorce into a nuclear format. After divorce a child still has two biological (nuclear) parents, although only one of these parents may be sharing a residence with the child. A basic requirement of the nuclear family model is that family members *must* share a residence, in order to be defined as such. Therefore, the biological parent who is not lived with is not included as part of a child's family; by definition this parent becomes "non-family" although the parent may or may not play an active part in the child's life.

A third problem in trying to superimpose the nuclear model onto the remarriage family, is that in remarriage families, the question arises as to whose perspective should be taken in defining family. This is a question that does not arise in the nuclear family because in almost all situations the children's kin are determined by parents' kin (adoption is an exception). A parent's mother is a child's maternal grandmother; a father's sister is an aunt, and so on. The parent's point of view is the one that is taken in defining family; it can automatically be assumed that parents' kin are also children's kin.

This taken-for-granted type of extended family structure does not exist for remarriage families. The parent remarried, and has a new spouse; but this new spouse is not a parent to the child, but rather, a stepparent. Also, the child's parents are in the relationship of ex-spouse to one another, although both are parents to the child. As well, there are all the kin related to the stepparent but not necessarily the child, and all the non-residential parent's kin related to the child but not to the co-residential parent (for example, a child's paternal grandparents are the mother's ex-in-laws).

In other words, the view of remarriage family structure is not the same for all participants. As Cherlin (1981) points out, definitions of family will vary from person to person due to the complex network of relationships created after divorce and remarriage. Therefore, in defining remarriage families, we must establish whose point of view we are taking and recognize this as one point of view among many.

The use of a subjective definition of family to establish the boundaries of remarriage families, allows us to go beyond the restrictions imposed by the nuclear model and to recognize one participant's point of view. It is the children's point of view which is expressed in this study, for two reasons.

The child's perspective has been neglected in family sociology (Skolnick and Skolnick, 1974; Eichler, 1983) and yet their structural position is crucial in a remarriage family. They are the connecting links between households—without them there would be no kinship overlap. If two adults remarry and neither of them have children from a previous marriage, the remarriage is similar in structure to a first marriage. Only when children are involved, is that new class of kin created, stepkin.

The purpose of this study was to develop a framework for analyzing remarriage families, which could take into account some of their properties without the need to copy or superimpose the nuclear family model onto them.

METHOD

This was an exploratory study, conducted in Toronto, Canada in 1982. The nonrandom sample consisted of sixty children, thirty males and thirty females, between the ages of sixteen and eighteen years old. The sample was obtained through advertisements and public service requests in local newspapers. In order to qualify as a respondent the following prerequisites were established: children were to have two living divorced parents, at least one of whom had a legal remarriage; and the child had to live with one of the biological parents, but not necessarily a remarried parent.

Of sixty children, fifty-two had one remarried parent and eight children, two. Thirty-five of the sixty children lived with a remarried parent, while twenty-five lived with an unmarried parent. These twenty-five had non-residential parents who were remarried. Forty-two children lived with their mothers, eighteen with their fathers.

A structured interview of approximately one hour was conducted. The children were asked whom they considered to be family members, as well as questions about their relationships with each of their biological parents and stepparents. The focus was the defining of family membership, the quality of their relationships as well as basic demographic information.

DEVELOPMENT OF A FRAMEWORK

Remarriage family structure was examined from the point of view of the children whose parents had remarried. The primary question was which of their parents, biological and step, did the children consider to be their family members, whether the children lived with them or not. In this way children had the option of including non-residential parents or stepparents as family members, as well as excluding co-residential parents and stepparents.

Parents were selected as the focus of family membership because "family" is traditionally defined in terms of parental membership, e.g., one-parent or two-parent family. This is not to say that siblings and other family are not important in defining family. It is just that using parental family membership allows comparisons to be made between traditional ways of defining remarriage family and those found in this study.

A typology was developed to categorize the choices that children could make with respect to parents in their remarriage family structure. This typology was based on the combination of parents the children included and excluded as family members. It is both mutually exclusive and exhaustive.

The framework theoretically differentiates respondents in a way that is personally meaningful to them. It also provides a vehicle for analyzing the remarriage family experiences of children and allows us to examine and combine disparate types of information.

Extensive exploratory data were collected, and from the data variables emerged which appeared to influence the child's placement within the typology. Patterns did occur, and those that applied to a majority of cases within each of the types are mentioned. Findings are briefly presented, somewhat tentatively due to the nonrandom sample and the small n's. They serve the purpose of breaking ground for further testing.

The names of the four types of family structure are retention, substitution, reduction and augmentation. The name of each type indicates the shift from the child's previous family structure i.e., prior to his or her parents' divorce. The assumption was made that in this previous family there were two parents, a mother and father, who were considered to be family members. Each of the four types will be described, as well as some of the characteristics of respondents within each type.

Retention

In retention are children in remarriage families who include both their biological parents as family members, the parent with whom they are living and the parent in a different household. A stepparent is not included as a family member.

This type makes us aware that it is possible to have a stepparent, even live with a stepparent, and not necessarily consider that person to be a family member. The children in this type "retain" their original two parents, and continue on identifying their families as they were prior to divorce and remarriage. The non-residential parent continues to be a family member, although he or she is no longer lived with.

This type is very different from the traditional view of remarriage family, as a stepparent is not incorporated into the children's subjective view of family membership. As well, a non-residential parent is not ignored. Children do not reconstruct their remarriage families as nuclear families, but rather hold on to the ties of their original nuclear families.

Twenty of the sixty respondents, i.e., thirty-three percent of the sample were found in retention. As we discovered from the data, the non-residential parent continued to play an important role in the life of the child. Visitation was frequent, and if infrequent due to distance, it was at least "future" oriented, i.e., a child may not have seen a parent "since last Christmas," but knew there would be a month's visitation during the summer holidays.

Sex was an important variable: sons more often included non-residential fathers as family members than did daughters. In fact same-sex loyalty appeared throughout all types in the study.

In most cases in retention the non-residential parent was a father. For over half the cases a child was living with a single mother, with a remarried father living in a different household. Many of these children had lived with their fathers at some time prior to the study, which could also help to account for their continued family ties with them. In fact approximately 30% of all children in the study at some point lived with the "other" non-residential parent.

Stepparents were not an important part of these children's lives, except in a negative way. Over half reported negative relationships with stepparents, and of those who liked their stepparents, feelings were not strong enough to include them as family members. Stepparents were seen as "outsiders" who "just weren't related."

One-third of the sample was found in retention, meaning that in spite of a parent moving out of the household and at least one parent remarrying, the children perceived *both* and *only* their original two parents as family members. Their definitions of family do not coincide with the traditional view of family as congruent with household membership.

Substitution

In substitution are children in remarriage families who exclude at least one biological parent and include at least one stepparent as family members. The most common example is the traditional view of the remarriage family, consisting of a child, remarried parent and his or her spouse.

The assumption is made in family sociology, taking marriage and family textbooks as an indication, that this type of remarriage family is a recreated nuclear family (Furstenberg, 1979). Mental health practitioners have recognized this for what it is, a myth. The myth assumes that stepparents and stepchildren form a family unit similar to that of biological parents and their children (Jacobson, 1979). In fact it has been found that belief in the myth negatively affects adjustment in remarriage families (Fast and Cain, 1966; Schulman, 1972; Jacobson, 1979).

Eight of the sixty respondents, or thirteen percent of the sample were in substitution. They included the biological parent and stepparent with whom they lived, and excluded the biological parent with whom they were not residing. For these children household and family membership were synonymous. How did these children perceive their parents and stepparents and does this fit in with the traditional view of remarriage family?

The eight respondents in substitution were living with a biological parent and stepparent, whom they included as family members, and had a biological parent living in a separate household. Again, sex could have been a factor as five of the eight respondents were females who included their stepfathers as family members, but not their non-residential fathers. Females accepted stepfathers more readily than did males in this study, and fathers in this type did not maintain regular or frequent contact with their daughters. The combination of these two factors could account for females including stepfathers and excluding fathers, in substitution.

All non-residential fathers had remarried or lived common-law with a person who had children. This has important implications as it has been found that men who have "new" families tend to have less involvement with the children from their first marriage as they give priority to the "new" children (Wallerstein and Kelly, 1980; Furstenberg and Spanier, 1984).

Respondents were younger at separation than those in the other types, and younger at remarriage. This increases the likelihood of a non-residential father fading from the child's life, and a stepparent becoming more involved.

The most interesting finding was that except in the case where a child was adopted by a stepfather, the stepparent although included as a family member, was still not totally regarded as a parent. There was always a qualification of the relationship, even though the stepparent was defined as "a parent" by the child. Statements were made such as "I really care about him, but I could never be as close to him as to my mother," or as another respondent said: "sometimes he takes on the father role, at other times he doesn't."

This is not surprising as Duberman (1975) reports similar findings. She found that "even those stepparents whose relationships with stepchildren were rated excellent could not completely fulfil the expectations of parent work." The finding is interesting for its contradiction of the traditional view of remarriage family, that a stepparent replaces a parent who no longer lives with the child. For the children in this study, even when they had a poor relationship with a non-residential parent and a good relationship with a stepparent, the stepparent was still not completely replacing a parent in all aspects of their lives.

Reduction

In reduction are those children in remarriage families who include fewer than their original two parents as family members. A stepparent is not identified as a family member, nor is at least one of their biological parents.

Theoretically, three situations are possible for children to qualify for this type: (1) neither parent is identified as a family member;

(2) the parent whom the child lives with is identified as a family member; or (3) the non-residential parent, is identified as a family member. All children in reduction in this study fulfilled the second situation: they identified the biological parent with whom they lived as a family member, excluding their non-residential parents and all stepparents.

Some respondents were actually living with stepparents, but did not include them as family members. Others were living with a single parent, and excluded their remarried non-residential parents and their spouses. There was a total of fifteen respondents in reduction, representing twenty-five percent of the sample.

The children who lived with a lone-parent whom they identified as their only parent, experienced family as a "one-parent family." This family type has been recognized, although the term is often applied erroneously to children who live with one parent yet have another parent with whom they identify, living elsewhere (Eichler, 1983). Children in retention who live with one parent would not consider themselves to be part of a "one-parent family."

Why might stepparents who are lived with be excluded as family members? Age at remarriage was very high for this group, and therefore remarriage had only occurred within a relatively short time prior to interview. Stepparents were not actively involved with the children in reduction, and most respondents reported negative feelings towards them.

Non-residential parents, mostly fathers, rarely saw their children in this type. Many respondents felt that they had been excluded by their fathers and new wives. Again, the majority of respondents in reduction were females who had a poor relationship with their non-residential fathers.

The respondents in reduction were, of all the children, the most dissatisfied with life and the most emotionally upset during the interviews. The denial of a second parent as a family member appeared to have taken a toll on their lives.

Augmentation

In augmentation are children in remarriage families who identify both their biological or first family parents as family member, as well as at least one stepparent. This type shares a tendency seen in recent studies to move away from the idea of a stepparent as a "replacement" and instead to see them as an "addition" to the family. This has been described in previous studies both implicitly and explicitly.

For example Furstenberg has explicitly recognized this principle of ''augmentation'' in his empirical work on remarriage, and in fact sees it as a positive benefit to the child because of access to more resources (Furstenberg and Spanier, 1984). He also reported that children were able to deal very well with this complexity, and ''seemed to be doing as well if not better in expanded family situations that in arrangements that involve the loss or replacement of a parent'' (Furstenberg and Nord, 1985)

Wallerstein and Kelly (1980) do not provide a label, but found that most of the children in their study who lived with stepfathers, enlarged their view of the family and made room for three major figures, mothers, stepfathers and non-residential fathers.

Theoretically, the expanded or augmented remarriage family does not exist; as well the literature suggests there are difficulties in establishing new ties with stepparents (Fast and Cain, 1966; Schlesinger and Stasiuk, 1972; McCormick, 1974; Messinger, 1976; Kompara, 1980; Lutz, 1983) as well as maintaining ties with the non-residential parent (Dominic and Schlesinger, 1980; Wallerstein and Kelly, 1980; Furstenberg et al., 1983; Palmer, 1983). What then characterizes the respondents in this study who were found in augmentation?

There were seventeen respondents in augmentation, or twenty-eight percent of the sample. Most respondents in augmentation lived with fathers and stepmothers. The fact that their non-residential parent was a mother could be a factor. Generally across types, it was found that mothers were more likely to maintain contact with their non-residential children than were fathers.

Also, fifty percent of respondents in augmentation had previously lived with their mothers, which may have accounted for a sustained relationship with her. Sex may have also been a factor, as the largest group in augmentation were males with stepmothers. If same-sex loyalty is a strong factor, which it appeared to be throughout the study, stepmothers and mothers could both be included by male respondents without fear of treason.

The children's median age at remarriage was average for the sample, but age at separation was high. This could also account for their continued relationship with non-residential parents.

All respondents in augmentation maintained contact with their non-residential parents, on a frequent or regular basis. There was a strong relationship with them, stronger than found in retention. Stepparents were mostly liked but were not seen as a replacement for the non-residential parent. The least positive relationships were between female respondents and stepmothers. Female respondents and stepfathers, male respondents and stepmothers generally had good relationships.

What specifically characterized respondents in augmentation was their freedom to move back and forth between households, and the apparent lack of hostility between their two biological parents and between a biological and stepparent of the same sex. Previous research has recognized that hostility between biological parents affects visitation with the non-residential parent (Fulton, 1979); Dominic and Schlesinger, 1980; Wallerstein and Kelly, 1980). Because of the lack of hostility the children were not forced to choose a parent over a stepparent or vice versa.

For these children family ties not only included but went beyond household membership. In this type, strong ties were maintained with both biological parents, and the stepparent was regarded as an addition to the family.

CONTRIBUTIONS AND CONCLUSIONS

The major contribution of this study is the development of a typology which is both mutually exclusive and exhaustive. The typology provides a conceptual framework which may be used to define types of remarriage families, from the child's perspective in a way that is directly meaningful to them. Also four configurations of remarriage families are recognized rather than assuming only the traditional remarriage family structure.

Theoretically the framework goes beyond the "deficit-comparison" approach in which any non-nuclear family is regarded as deficient in some aspect, because of its non-nuclear structure (Ganong and Coleman, 1984). Although the typology is based on the change or lack of change between the nuclear family parental structure and the child's perception of parental membership, remarriage families are not seen as deficient or lacking simply because of their non-nuclear structure.

Also, the framework goes beyond the "household = family" model which leaves out some family members and includes other just on the basis of shared residence. A family is not contained within walls. Family may be more or less than household membership, a fact fully recognized in this study.

Several variables are suggested which may contribute to the child's placement within the typology. Some of these are: co-residence and prior co-residence; age at separation and remarriage as well as time since separation and remarriage; remarriage and additional children of a non-residential parent; sex of respondent, stepparent and non-residential parent; visitation with non-residential parent; and quality of relationships.

Due to the small, non-random sample these descriptions are only just that: exploratory and suggestive. The effects of these cannot be generalized to a larger population of children in remarriage families, but there influence could be tested in a large-scale study with a random sample. It would also be interesting to include siblings—biological, half and step—to see their configuration within remarriage family structure.

An additional contribution of this study is discovering what children themselves have to say about family structure. The perspectives of family theorists, and the perspectives of children experiencing remarriage families obviously do not necessarily coincide. The children's point of view should be taken into account much more frequently in matters such as these, which impinge on them so directly.

This framework can be a starting point for further analyzing child-parent relationships in remarriage families, from the child's perspective. It goes beyond the assumptions of household = family, stepparent as parent, and remarriage family as recreated nuclear family. Such assumptions have impeded the study of remarriage families because they have not taken into account the realities of the experiences of family members.

REFERENCES

Bohannan, P. (1971). Divorce chains, households of remarriage, and multiple divorcers. In P. Bohannan (Ed.), *Divorce and After* (pp. 127–139). New York: Doubleday.

Bumpass, L. (1984). Some characteristics of children's second families. *American Journal of Sociology, 90*(3), 608–623.

Cherlin, A. (1981). *Marriage, Divorce, Remarriage*. Cambridge, MA: Harvard University Press.

Dominic, K. T., & Schlesinger, B. (1981). Weekend fathers: family shadows. *Journal of Divorce 3*(3), 241–247.

Duberman, L. (1975). *The Reconstituted Family*. Chicago: Nelson-Hall.

Eichler, M. (1983). *Families in Canada Today: Recent Changes and Their Policy Consequences*. Toronto: Gage.

Esses, L. & Campbell, R. (1984). Challenges in researching the remarried. *Family Relations 33*(3), 415–424.

Fast, I. & Cain A. C. (1966). The stepparent role: potential for disturbances in family functioning. *American Journal of Orthopsychiatry 36*(3), 485–491.

Fulton, J. A. (1979). Parental reports of children's post-divorce adjustment. *Journal of Social Issues 35*(4), 126–139.

Furstenberg, F. F., Jr. (1979). Recycling the family: perspectives for a neglected family form. *Marriage and Family Review 2*(3), 1, 12–22.

Furstenberg, F. F., Jr., Nord, C. W., Peterson, J. L., & Zill, N. (1983). The life course of children of divorce. *American Sociological Review 48*(5), 656–668.

Furstenberg, F. F., Jr., & Spanier, G. B. (1984). *Recycling the Family*. Beverly Hills, CA: Sage.

Ganong, L. H., & Coleman, M. (1984). The effects of remarriage on children: a review of the empirical literature. *Family Relations 33*(3), 389–406.

Jacobson, D. (1979). Stepfamilies: myths and realities. *Social Work 24*(3), 202–207.

Kompara, D. R. (1980). Difficulties in the socialization process of stepparenting. *Family Relations 29*(1), 69–73.

Lutz, P. (1983). The stepfamily: an adolescent perspective. *Family Relations 32*(3), 367–375.

McCormick, M. (1974). *Stepfathers: What the Literature Reveals*. Western Behavioral Sciences Institute: La Jolla, CA.

Messinger, L. (1976). Remarriage between divorced people with children from previous marriages: A proposal for preparation for remarriage. *Journal of Marriage and Family Counseling 2*(2), 193–200.

Messinger, L., Walker, K. N., & Freeman, S. J. J. (1978). Preparation for remarriage following divorce: The use of Group Techniques. *American Journal of Orthopsychiatry 48*(2), 263–272.

Palmer, S. (1983). The initial effect of divorce upon children. In K. Ishwaran (Ed.), *Marriage and Divorce in Canada* (pp. 297–326). Toronto, Canada: Methuen.

Price-Bonham, S., & Balswick, J. O. (1980). The noninstitutions: divorce, desertion and remarriage. *Journal of Marriage and the Family 42*(4), 959–972.

Sager, D. J., Brown, H. S., Crohn, H., Engel, T., Rodstein, E., & Walker, L. (1983). *Treating the Remarriage Family*. New York: Brunner/Mazel.

Schlesinger, B. & Stasiuk, E. (1972). Children of divorced parents in second marriages. In I. R. Stuart & L. E. Abt (Eds.), *Children of Separation and Divorce* (pp.19–35). New York: Grossman.

Schneider, D. M. (1980). *American Kinship: A Cultural Account*. Chicago: University of Chicago Press.

Schulman, G. L. (1972). Myths that intrude on the adaptation of the stepfamily. *Social Casework 53*(3), 131–139.

Skolnick, A. & Skolnick, J. H. (1974). *Intimacy, Family and Society*. Boston: Little, Brown & Co.

Statistics Canada. (1983). *Divorce: Law and the Family in Canada*. Ottawa: Minister of Supply and Services.

Wallerstein, J. S. & Kelly, J. B. (1980). *Surviving the Breakup*. New York: Basic Books.

GROUP TREATMENT MODELS FOR DIVORCING POPULATIONS

The Long-Term Effects of Divorce: Mothers and Children in Concurrent Support Groups

Ana Margarita Cebollero
Karen Cruise
Gary Stollak

ABSTRACT. Supportive services in the form of concurrent groups for mothers and children experiencing the long-term negative effects of divorce are described. The general goal of the Single Parent Project was to provide parents and children an environment within which they could experience a cohesive feeling of support and sharing, and the opportunity to learn new communication and problem-solving skills. Each group (parent and child) was run by a graduate student. Clinical supervision was conjoint, helping to maintain conceptual unity of each family system. Issues presented by mothers or children were used to develop strategies for subsequent meetings. Although this project explored the effectiveness of a variety of interventions, two deserve special mention: (1) All siblings aged 4 through 12 were included, with no identification of a problem child. (2) Mothers served as co-therapists in the children's group. Problems inherent in a pilot study of this nature are discussed. A

Gary Stollak, PhD, is Professor, Department of Psychology, Michigan State University. Ana Margarita Cebollero and Karen Cruise are graduate students in that program. Correspondence regarding this article may be addressed to Gary Stollak, Department of Psychology, Michigan State University, Psychology Research Building, East Lansing, MI 48824.

primary benefit to both groups was social support and a decrease in social isolation.

An increasing number of people have sought counseling to help them deal with the process of post-divorce adjustment and change. Services provided for men and women have included individual therapy (Wallerstein & Kelly, 1977), structured, short-term group treatment (Granvold & Welch, 1979; Stolberg & Garrison, 1985; Warren & Amara, 1985), educational workshops (Rugel & Sieracki, 1981), and single-parent support groups (Jauch, 1977). These services have focused on issues of interpersonal competency (Magid, 1977), maintenance of emotional and social adjustment (Pett, 1982), and the effects of divorce on children (Hetherington, Cox & Cox, 1978).

Services have also been provided in a variety of settings to meet the needs of the children. Interventions found most effective with preschool children are generally those made on their behalf through the parents over a prolonged period of time (Gardner, 1977; Wallerstein & Kelly, 1975). For the early school-aged child, intervention seems most easily facilitated through dialogues which enable the child to see that other children his/her age have similar problems and feelings (Kelly & Wallerstein, 1977). In later childhood and preadolescence, maturity and greater cognitive and linguistic skills allow greater variety of direct interventions. These children benefit from reassurance and reality-testing with the therapist, and encouragement to raise the same issues with their parents (Kelly & Wallerstein, 1977; Rohrlich, Ranier, Berg-Cross & Berg-Cross, 1977; Stolberg & Garrison, 1985).

There has also been increasing interest both in the use of groups for delivery of services to children of divorce and in provision of these services outside of a clinical setting. Such programs are designed to meet the needs of a much larger population of children who can be seen as needing certain services based solely on their parents' marital status. Scheidlinger (1984) differentiated such services from those commonly referred to as "therapy," calling them "therapeutic." He also expressed the hope that therapeutic services delivered in a group setting will help children to cope better with this shared life-stress and prevent the development of severe psychopathology.

In order to reach as many children as possible, group interventions have increasingly taken place in schools (Campbell, 1984, Cantor, 1977; Hammond, 1981; Kalter, Pickar, Lesowitz, 1984; Sonnenshein-Schneider & Baird, 1980) and the community at large (Guerney & Jordan, 1979; Kessler & Bostwick, 1977; Magid, 1977). These groups have varied in time frame, ages of children, general format and structure. Goals for these groups, however, have consistently been to provide the child with support, emotional catharsis, and information. The groups facilitate interaction with peers experiencing similar difficulties, assist the child in gaining a realistic view of divorce, and provide an opportunity to understand and express feelings and develop and enhance coping strategies. Preliminary evaluations suggest that these groups have been successful in impacting the child's adjustment to divorce (Kessler & Bostwick, 1977).

The groups described above have primarily served parents and children currently or recently involved in divorce. The project described herein was designed to provide supportive or therapeutic services for families for whom divorce had occurred two or more years ago, and for whom the initial critical stage of adjustment, hopefully, had passed. The initial model was modified to fit the needs presented by the mothers and their children as the group proceeded.

THE SINGLE PARENT PROJECT

Project Objectives

The general goal of the Single Parent Project was to provide parents and children an environment within which they could experience a cohesive feeling of support and sharing, and the opportunity to learn new communication skills and problem-solving strategies. Specific therapeutic goals of the women's group included exploration of assumptions and feelings about marriage, divorce, and single parenthood. Specific goals for the children were discussion of thoughts and feelings about the divorce and their present lives.

Recruitment

The project was advertised through local newspapers, clergymen, Friend of the Court, and the university Psychological clinic where the group meetings were held. It is important to note that the project was initially intended to serve both single parent men and women. One man expressed interest but did not attend. A total of twenty-two women inquired about the group. Of these, eleven were seeking services not provided by the group. The children's group was concurrently established and attendance of all children aged four and older in each family was encouraged. Four of the women decided against attending because their adolescent male children refused participation.

Composition

The women's group was comprised of the remaining seven women, who ranged in age from 29 to 37 (Mean age = 33). One of these women had taken some college courses, four were current college students, one had a bachelor's degree, and one, a master's degree. All of the women had custody of their children. Mean number of children per family was 2.9. Time lapsed since the divorce ranged from 2 to 4 years.

A total of fifteen children, ranging in age from 4 through 12 (mean age = 7.3), attended the children's group over the course of project. A core group of seven children attended most of the sessions. These children were aged 5 through 10, with a mean age of 6.7 years.

Structure

The women and children were involved in an intake, weekly 1–1/2 hour group sessions (twenty weeks for the women, seventeen for the children), a termination session, and a follow-up home visit at four months. Groups were kept open to new members for the first ten weeks. Participants were charged a fee according to their financial resources. Child care was provided free of charge to families having children under age four. Information gathered at the intake included presenting problems, an informal assessment of intellectual and emotional functioning of the mother, and mother and child reports of the children's perceptions about living in a single parent family and their general adjustment.

Each of the two groups (parent and child) was run by a female graduate student in her 40's. Clinical supervision was conjoint, helping to maintain conceptual unity of each family system. The role of the therapist was directive, using different therapeutic strategies to create change. Two of these strategies deserve special mention: (1) All age-appropriate siblings were included, with no identification of a problem child. (2) Mothers served as co-therapists in the children's group. Issues presented by mothers (e.g., excessive crying) or children (e.g., visitation problems) were used to develop agendas for subsequent meetings.

Group Activities: Adults

The interventions utilized in the women's group included group discussion, homework, written meeting summaries, and processing of mother's involvement in the children's group as co-therapists. The mothers and children spent an early joint session becoming acquainted. At a later point in time, the mothers conducted one session of the women's group without a therapist present.

These women lead hectic lives, involving many responsibilities and financial stresses. Almost all of them had experienced severe conflict prior to their divorce. In some cases, this conflict took the form of incest and/or abuse. Children were a basic concern, with problems in parenting frequently revolving around inconsistency in responding to the behaviors of the children. Some of the women responded to a fear of losing control of their children and themselves through excessively authoritarian and punishing behaviors; others responded by submitting and allowing their children to engage in unacceptable behaviors. Many experienced taking care of their children as overwhelming. They discussed their children's school problems and the children's relationships with their fathers. They talked at length about their children's behaviors. All of the women experienced difficulty in responding to their children's expressions of anger and sadness. Another recurring theme was the women's sense that they would have to wait for their children to grow up before they could pursue their own interests. One woman, after discussing with the group her desire to remarry her second husband against her children's wishes, announced her decision in favor of the remarriage and stopped attending meetings. A follow-up telephone call confirmed her continuing plans to remarry and move to another state.

All of the women were experiencing financial stresses. Even the college graduates who had jobs were struggling to provide for their children. Two of the women were in extremely precarious financial situations, which imposed limitations on their exploration of alternatives for housing and transportation. They experienced difficulties related to work and school. While in the group, one woman dropped out of school, and another had a full-time position cut to half time. She is now working two part-time jobs. These experiences are consistent with the literature, which indicates that economic problems in single parent women are related to significantly higher levels of stress (Colletta, 1983).

A pervasive sense of loneliness and the need to engage in social and sexually intimate relationships were extensively discussed in the women's group. The women both desired and were still uncomfortable with offers of male companionship. Single parent women can be significantly affected by loneliness and isolation in social situations even two or more years post-divorce (see also Woodward, Zabel & Decosta, 1980). The majority of these women placed their children's concerns first, and were afraid the children would experience difficulties if they remarried. In a particularly poignant session where intimacy and sexuality were discussed, one of the women revealed that she was pregnant.

The women consistently reported having "nobody to talk to who could understand" what their lives were like. The support the women provided to each other, most notably in crisis and emergency situations, was incredible, and extended, with time, beyond the confines of the group setting. There was pleasure in each other's company and much laughter. Small achievements were applauded. One of the women underwent corrective breast surgery. During the next meeting, for the first time, she did not wear a coat. Her happiness was everyone's joy. At the same time, it was especially difficult for group members to deal with angry feelings toward each other, and learning to give feedback was continually problematic and painful.

As termination approached, the women expressed a wish to continue meeting. One woman referred to her experience in the group as "like having money in the bank . . . I might need to draw from it someday."

Group Activities: Children

The children's group was loosely structured to include group activities, discussion (circle time), and free play. Group activities included drawings by the children of themselves and their families, puppet shows, and games. During one session, older and younger children worked together in triads drawing self-portraits and listing feelings and other words which described themselves. During circle time, children were encouraged to talk about their feelings. Topics included discussions of what various family members did that made the children feel happy, angry or sad, and what the children could do with those feelings. The children talked about their parent's divorce, what they imagined would happen if their parents were married again, and how it feels to tell friends their parents are divorced.

The open group structure resulted in several sessions devoted to incorporating new members into the group. Despite this potential disruption, however, the group remained both cohesive and flexible. Because of the number of children and their age span, it was often difficult to engage all of the children in similar activities. On several occasions, the group was divided into younger and older children. This facilitated group discussions, but the children were reluctant to be separated. It became increasingly clear that the children as a larger group functioned as support for each other. As one of the older children described it, the group felt like "a family."

Involving mothers who alternated as co-leaders in the children's group was highly successful. Each child was delighted with his/her mother's presence, and participation of all of the children in group and circle activities was facilitated. The presence of the mother did not inhibit sharing of feelings, as might have been expected. This may have been a feature of introducing co-therapy after the group had been in process for a number of weeks, rather than at the outset. This openness can be illustrated by one group interaction involving discussion of what made the children sad about their parent's divorce. One co-leader mother stated that she was sad that she couldn't provide the kind of family she thought her children should have. One of her children said she sometimes thought that if she hadn't been born, her parents would not have divorce.

Occasional difficulties were encountered as a result of aggressive acting out by the children. Sporadic episodes of aggressive behavior coincided with custody problems, parental dating, and problems with living arrangements reported by the mothers. The children's functioning in the group clearly varied by developmental level. The younger children enjoyed the group activities and social interaction. They were able to identify global feelings discussed in circle but, with some exceptions, were more limited in talking about their own feelings than were the older children. Some of the children expressed a sense of being different from other children, and limited in their friendships. Anger and sadness related to parental divorce were expressed by all of the children. Children who had been very young at the time of the divorce talked about missing their fathers and wishing their parents were still married. A discussion of what the children thought would happen if their parents were married again brought different reactions from the older children, however. They expressed concerns about parental arguing and fighting, and recalled their own unhappiness during the time of the divorce. These children did not want reconciliation. The children also talked about their current relationships with each parent, and most expressed satisfaction with their living arrangments. Children who saw their fathers regularly reported feeling good about that relationship. One child expressed hurt and anger at unanswered letters and unobserved birthdays.

Overall, the group provided a place where the children could discuss their feelings and talk with and become friends with other children who had similar feelings and life experiences. Children whose mothers began seeing each other outside of the group expressed pleasure with these new relationships.

DISCUSSION

It was apparent that although the divorce for these women and children was two years or more in the past, they were still struggling with the long-range effects of this event. This observation is consistent with the results of research which indicate that the crisis of divorce might extend well beyond two years and that this factor must be considered in the planning of interventions (Felner, Farber, Ginter, Boike & Cowen, 1981). In the project described above, both women and children were given an opportunity to discuss the feelings, thoughts, and needs resulting from their common experience. Their reactions appear to indicate that a primary benefit to both groups was social support and the resulting decrease of social isolation.

Development of format on a week-to-week basis facilitated the ability of this project to meet the individual needs of these women and children. It also required expenditure of considerable therapist time. The use of a closed group format would have resulted in a more stable structure and the potential for greater predictability related to these needs, thereby reducing the time required for planning.

The decision to include all preadolescent siblings of interested mothers resulted in a children's group of frequently unmanageable size. The need for more than one therapist was immediately apparent. Although involvement of parents as co-therapists helped to meet this need, the therapeutic nature of this intervention would have been facilitated either by use of more than one core therapist or by training of the co-therapist parent. The alternative of limiting the number of children would have meant participation of fewer parents. In this project, this would have precluded the use of mothers as co-therapists, as the mothers group would often have been too small. Further limitation of age range of siblings included in the children's group would have been another possible alternative.

REFERENCES

Campbell, C. (1984, August). *Impact of group counseling on primary school children of divorce*. Paper presented at the 92nd annual convention of the American Psychological Association at Toronto, Ontario, Canada.

Cantor, D. (1977). School-based groups for children of divorce. *Journal of Divorce, 1*(2), 183–187.

Colletta, N. (1983). Stressful lives: The situation of divorced mothers and their children. *Journal of Divorce, 6*(3), 19–31.

Felner, R., Farber, S., Ginter, M., Boike, M. & Cowen, E. (1981). Family stress and organization following parental divorce or death. *Journal of Divorce, 4*(2), 67–76.

Gardner, R. (1977). Children of divorce—some legal and psychological considerations. *Journal of Clinical Child Psychology, 6*(2), 3–6.

Granvold, D. K. & Welch, G. J. (1979). Structured, short-term group treatment of postdivorce adjustment. *International Journal of Group Psychotherapy, 29*(4), 347–357.

Guerney, L. & Jordan, L. (1979). Children of divorce—A community support group. *Journal of Divorce, 2*(3), 283–294.

Hammond, J. (1981). Loss of the family unit: Counseling groups to help kids. *The Personnel and Guidance Journal, 59*(2), 392–394.

Hetherington, E., Cox, M. & Cox, M. (1978). The aftermath of divorce. In J. H. Stevens, Jr. & M. Mathews (Eds.), *Mother/Child/Father/Child Relationships*, pp. 149–176. Washington, D. C.: National Association for the Education of Young Children.

Jauch, J. (1977). The one-parent family. *Journal of Clinical Child Psychology, 6*(2), 30–32.

Kalter, N., Pickar, J. & Lesowitz, M. (1984). School based developmental facilitation groups for children of divorce: A preventive intervention. *American Journal of Orthopsychiatry, 54*(4), 613–623.

Kelly, J. & Wallerstein, J. (1977). Brief intervention with children in divorce families. *American Journal of Orthopsychiatry, 47*(1), 23–39.

Kessler, S. & Bostwick, S. (1977). Beyond divorce: Coping skills for children. *Journal of Clinical Child Psychology, 6*(2), 38–41.

Magid, K. (1977). Children facing divorce: A treatment program. *Personnel and Guidance Journal, 55*(9), 534–536.

Pett, M. (1982). Correlates of children's social adjustment following divorce. *Journal of Divorce, 5*(4), 25–39.

Rohrlich, J., Ranier, R., Berg-Cross, L. & Berg-Cross, G. (1977). The effects of divorce: A research review with a developmental perspective. *Journal of Clinical Child Psychology, 6*(2), 15–20.

Rugel, R. P. & Sieracki, S. (1981). The single parent workshop: An approach to the problem of children of divorce. *Journal of Clinical Child Psychology, 10*(3), 159–164.

Scheidlinger, S. (1984). Short-term group psychotherapy for children: An overview. *International Journal of Group Psychotherapy, 34*(4), 573–585.

Sonnenshein-Schneider, M. & Baird, K. (1980). Group counseling children of divorce in the elementary schools: Understanding process and technique. *The Personnel and Guidance Journal, 59*(2), 88–91.

Stolberg, A. L., & Garrison, K. M. (1985). Evaluating a primary prevention program for children of divorce. *American Journal of Community Psychology, 13*(2), 111–124.

Wallerstein, J. (1978, November). *The effects of divorce on the parent-child relationship.* Paper presented at the Symposium on Children and Divorce, Wheelock College, Boston, Massachusetts.

Wallerstein, J. S. & Kelly, J. B. (1975). The effects of parental divorce: Experiences of the preschool child. *Journal of the American Academy of Child Psychiatry, 14*, 600–616.

Wallerstein, J. S. & Kelly, J. B. (1976). The effects of parental divorce: Experiences of the child in later latency. *American Journal of Orthopsychiatry, 46*(2), 256–269.

Wallerstein, J. S. & Kelly, J. B. (1977). Divorce counseling: A community service for families in the midst of divorce. *American Journal of Orthopsychiatry, 47*(1), 4–22.

Warren, N. J., & Amara, I. A. (1985). Educational groups for single parents: The parenting after divorce programs. *Journal of Divorce, 8*(2), 79–96.

Woodward, J., Zabel, J. & DeCosta, C. (1980). Loneliness and divorce. *Journal of Divorce, 4*(1), 73–83.

Group Work with Emotionally Attached or Ambivalent Spouses in Process of Separating, Separated, or Recently Divorced

Roxanne Power

ABSTRACT. This paper addresses the specific needs of a clearly delineated population of individuals who are finding difficulty adjusting to the irrevocable, but often unwanted, loss of a partner through separation or divorce. A description of an emotionally attached or ambivalent person is presented as well as the intrapsychic and interpersonal problems they experience which impede the cognitive, emotional and behavioral adjustments they must make. The group is discussed in terms of composition, goals, interventive strategies, and role of the therapist.

Divorce is a rapidly growing phenomena in North America. At least 40% of Canadian marriages now end in divorce (Statistics Canada, 1983) while similar statistics in the United States further highlight the seriousness of this problem. The aftermath affects not only the marital couple but also their offspring who may suffer unwanted separation from a parent, as well as the families of origin who frequently offer emotional, economic, or housing supports.

Divorce has been defined as

> . . . a social, emotional, and legal process through which the former spouses come to regard themselves and be regarded by others, as single individuals. . . . Divorce can also be viewed as a transition process bridging marriage and another lifestyle. (Brown, 1976a, p. 2)

Roxanne Power is a PhD candidate at the School of Social Work, University of Toronto, Canada. This paper was presented at the Seventh Annual Symposium of Social Group Workers, New Jersey, October 1985.

Before one can emotionally accept divorce or separation and begin an individualization process, a wide range of responses may be experienced including anger, denial, depression, ambivalence, and guilt (Brown et al., 1980; Nass, 1977).

Although several theories have been proposed to explain why people divorce (e.g., Goode, 1966; Levinger, 1965; Moles & Levinger, 1976), Weiss explained an alternate perspective. He (1975) studied why some people refuse to consider a divorce alternative or do not adjust successfully after its occurrence. His conclusions led to a proposed theory of emotional attachment or ambivalence to explain the psychological insecurity and dependency which makes some people reluctant to separate or adjust successfully.

The remainder of this paper will address how group work may stabilize the dramatic effect that pending or actual divorce or separation has on the emotionally attached or ambivalent spouse in the realms of intrapsychic and interpersonal functioning. Issues of identification of an emotionally attached or ambivalent spouse, group composition, focus of work, and leader role will be discussed.

WHO IS EMOTIONALLY ATTACHED OR AMBIVALENT?

Identification of an emotionally attached or ambivalent spouse is a prime concern in problem assessment and planned intervention. Weiss (1975) defined emotional attachment as a bonding to the other which permits " . . . feelings of at-homeness and ease when the other is present, or if not present, is felt to be accessible" (p. 304). These feelings of ease may be interrupted with periods of marital confrontation, but yet the emotionally attached spouse may prefer frequent negative spousal interaction (e.g., arguments or nonharmonious silence) to a separation or divorce alternative.

Often divorce is not a mutual decision (Cuber & Harroff, 1965; Kressel, 1980; Weiss, 1975) and the spouse initiating divorce may have been secretly contemplating this decision for several months before any definitive action was taken (Goode, 1956). The noninitiating spouse with less time to adjust to the pending divorce may be emotionally unready to cope with this reality (Brown, 1976b; Kressel et al., 1980). The response of the less emotionally prepared spouse may be continued emotional attachment to the spouse long after the divorce (Brown et al., 1980; Kitson, 1982; Weiss, 1975).

Evidence of such an attachment may take the forms of refusal to consider or plan for a pending divorce, efforts to delay the divorce through numerous property or child custody battles, frequent preoccupation with the past, seeking unnecessary interactions with the absent partner, and reluctance to engage in activities that mark a transition to single status (e.g., social participation, taking a role formerly assumed by spouse).

Ambivalence has been described by Marris (1974) as desiring to

> . . . consolidate all that is still valuable and important in the past, and preserve it from loss; and at the same time, to re-establish a meaningful pattern of relationships, in which the loss is accepted (p. 31).

Thus, the ambivalent spouse or couple vacillates between separation and reunion. There is recognition that a problem exists coupled with a reluctance to finalize any decisions; hence, no meaningful effort is made to resolve the problem.[1] The ambivalent spouse may exhibit difficulty reaching a final decision regarding a permanent separation or divorce, or once having finalized the legal process may admit doubts about the wisdom of the action.

Several factors may influence the presence and degree of emotional attachment or ambivalence. Sudden separations permit less time for the non-initiator to emotionally accept the reality of the situation (Spanier & Casto, 1979; Zeiss et al., 1980). Further, the length of marriage may contribute to the degree of emotional distress experienced following separation. Brown et al. (1980) and Weiss (1975) found that separation from any marriage of longer than two years duration was emotionally distressful, while others have found that short marriages result in less emotional distress upon separation (Hetherington et al., 1978; Kurdek & Blisk, 1983; Raschke, 1977). As well, those spouses who separated marital/parental roles according to gender or personal preference or who engaged primarily in conjoint social activities and mostly communal friends may experience more emotional ambivalence in their post-separation experience (Spanier & Casto, 1979; Weiss, 1975).

A summary of the emotional and cognitive intrapsychic responses to emotional acceptance/non-acceptance of separation or divorce is illustrated in Figure 1 (Power, in press). Regardless of initial presenting problem, clients contemplating divorce or those recently separated or divorced who fit any of the above categories or

I. Intrapsychic - Cognitive/Emotional

Acceptance

Intrapsychic

- Accept "separation is for best"
- Tentative plans for future
- Loneliness in general
- Realistic Anxiety for future
- Infrequent thoughts of spouse
- Rational, calm action
- Appropriate mood affect
- "The marriage is ended"
- As initiator you feel you have "done the right thing"
- As recipient you feel you must accept the situation; "make the best of it"
- Perceiving the need to separate

Non-Acceptance

- "Maybe we should try again"; ambivalence
- Excessive rumination with past
- Loneliness for spouse
- Feelings of "can't cope alone"
- Preoccupation with thinking about spouse
- Impulsiveness; poor judgment
- High intensity of feelings and mood fluctuations
- "We've separated before". This is temporary
- As initiator you feel guilty; selfish
- As recipient you feel rejection; hurt; anger
- Cognitive dissonance (e.g. using kids, poor health, etc. to stay together)

FIGURE 1

who exhibit dysfunctional thinking or affect as noted below, should be carefully assessed regarding their emotional readiness to accept the finality of the marital dissolution.

Individuals who remain emotionally attached to their separated or ex-spousal partners, or who are ambivalent about the divorce itself, may experience difficulties in the various process of divorce which Bohannon (1970) has labelled as legal, economic, co-parenting, community, and psychic phases. The focus of group work addressed later in this paper is an effort to enhance adjustment in these three latter spheres of interpersonal (i.e., co-parenting and community) and intra-personal functioning.

GROUP COMPOSITION

Group work with the emotionally attached or ambivalent spouse optimally should include a mixture of male and female persons who are currently separated, recently divorced (i.e., within past 18 months), or those presently living together but seriously contemplating marital disengagement. This group composition allows a more comprehensive overview of the different phases of inner emotional responses and external behavioral activities that each stage of uncoupling encompasses. Thus, the member contemplating separation can learn of the future positive potential and hazards experienced by the separated and divorced counterparts. Members can transfer to others their knowledge of progression along a road to eventual acceptance and adjustment. As well, they can learn to recognize that their overwhelming fears of existence without a partner are irrational, but common, reactions to separation and divorce. Yalom (1975) noted that the curative factors of instillation of hope, altruism, and universality are highly valued by group members.

FOCUS OF GROUP WORK

The integral components of successful divorce adjustment include emotional acceptance of the divorce and restructuring of lifestyle (Spanier & Casto, 1979; Sprenkle & Storm, 1982). A summary of the restructuring tasks are outlined in Figure 2 (Power, in press) and revolve around assuming new roles in dyadic interac-

II.

Restructuring Tasks	Possible Blocks to Restructuring
A. Marital Dyad Interaction	
- Conflict is situational - focused	- Conflict is person-focused; used to maintain relationship
- Appropriate pattern of interaction with spouse	- Frequent, unnecessary contact with spouse
- Moderate/low intensity of conflict	- High intensity of conflict
- Respect for spouse's decision to separate	- Use of coercion or emotional appeals to reunite
- Redistribution of marital tasks	- Reluctance to change status quo
- Effort toward conflict resolution	- Issue avoidance; conflict escalation; need to "save face"
- Beginning to integrate new life-style	- Inability to handle routine of new way of life
B. Interaction with Children	
- Children informed of marital decision and its impact on them	- Minimal or negative reference of separation made to kids
- Children encouraged to remain close to both parents	- Children encouraged to take sides
- Children's time with each parent is respected	- Plans often changed; children used as "spies" and "messengers"
- Maintaining appropriate parental child interaction	- Excessive time spent with kids; child used as "therapist" for parent

FIGURE 2

- Each parent has agreed parental tasks for all kids and/or each child	- Efforts to "block" other parent's actions; dysfunction coalitions
C. <u>Significant Others</u>	
- Separation explained to others	- Minimal/no discussion with others
- Engage in activities outside home	- Little interest in outside activities
- Support of family, friends, etc.	- Infrequent/inappropriate use of support

FIGURE 2, continued

tion in a now defunct marital union, interaction with offspring and significant others (e.g., family of origin, friends, social agencies).

The restructuring tasks of life as a single person and parent within these three different realms occur simultaneously, and hence a tremendous amount of psychic and physical energy is required to adapt successfully to new roles. Emotional attachment or ambivalence in a separated or divorced spouse may hinder or prolong successful completion of these restructuring tasks which Brown (1976b) and Weiss (1975) have stated may normally take one to two years before a person can cope comfortably alone.

TASK OF GROUP WORK

The main tasks or activity in the working phase of the group's development should center around resolution of these key areas of emotional acceptance and restructuring. Knowledge of how members subjectively perceive their own functioning and how they are objectively functioning should give the therapist some insights for positive intervention. The objective assessment may arise from direct observation of the member in the group, feedback from the member and significant others (e.g., professional staff, family), and other members' in-group perceptions and comments. Figure 3 helps to illustrate how prior knowledge of the common problems in this population coupled with knowledge of the individual members' functioning level may help the therapist anticipate appropriate intervention.

It must be cautioned, however, that problem-solving in the working phase is not the sole responsibility of the therapist. Members should be encouraged to actively help another member through sharing personal solutions to similar problems or offering other tentative suggestions. Similarly, the therapist and members should regularly check back with other members to see what problem-solving actions were tried and the consequent results.

THERAPIST'S ROLE

The group therapist's position should be more of a facilitator and expert consultant. These members already suffer from emotional attachment or ambivalence and hence they should not be encouraged to transfer this dependency to a perceived authoritarian or protective

Possible Task Focus in the Group Working Phase

ANTICIPATED PROBLEM	PROBLEM-SOLVING SUGGESTIONS
members' excessive rumination of past when alone	(a) have member spend equal time contemplating the negatives of marriage and spouse's faults
members' excessive discussion of past in group session	(a) set ground rules that all group discussion should primarily be present-focused (b) stress problem-solving of current problems, not analysis of past
personal feelings of rejection, worthlessness, guilt, etc.	(a) have member list their own positive attributes (aloud or alone) (b) have group members contribute to the list or give feed-back (c) ask members if this is a common reaction shared by others present (d) emphasize the normalcy of these feelings
inability to discuss separation with parents, children, neigh-bours, etc.	(a) have members rehearse in the group what they would like to say and receive constructive feedback (b) help them pick a most appropriate time and place for discussion
reluctance to engage in activities alone outside the home	(a) self-preparation of a list of preferred social activities (b) confirm one activity they could do during the week (c) have them anticipate problems which may occur and how to handle these (e.g. what if no one wants to talk to me, what to tell my kids if they ask where I am going?) (d) arrange a buddy to accompany them initially, if necessary
initiating frequent unnecessary contact with absent spouse	(a) set a definite appropriate time to call weekly/bi-monthly etc. about conjoint items (b) prepare a list in advance to avoid forgetting and hence extra calls

FIGURE 3

figure. Realistically in the beginning the therapist may need to assume a more directive approach, e.g., taking more responsibility for informal agenda-setting, offering ideas for group discussion, role modeling appropriate self-disclosure, and eliciting members' input. However, this type of group has a great deal of emotional energy because of the crisis period, and this may constitute a mitigating variable (Lang, 1979) which acts to hasten group feelings of cohesion, sharing, and mutual problem-solving. Certainly the worker should make frequent references to the ability of members to solve their own dilemmas with solicited input from other group participants who have encountered similar problems.

Co-leadership by male and female therapists may help to ease the emotional tension of both participant sexes. Co-leaders can role model how differences of opinion can be positively negotiated, while exposing male and female members to cross gender emotional viewpoints on divorce. If only one therapist is available to lead the group, care must be taken to ensure that a conscious/unconscious personal bias is not present in the therapists group approach (e.g., women make the best parents; non-initiators are victims).

In addition to the dilemmas of dependency transference or sexual biasing the therapist(s) must be alert to the possibility of premature or "rebound" romantic attractions between members who are in very vulnerable emotional states. There are several precautions a worker may take to prevent this, including a prearranged seating rotation, changing discussion group compositions, and planning activities which encourage active involvement among all members. When mutual attractions do occur the group should be helped to comfortably discuss the situation openly and positively. The naturalness of this event should be emphasized and the situation used as a forum for general discussion of issues such as how to relate to a new dating partner, how to handle familiar social gatherings with a new partner, and the fear of personal inadequacies or another rejection. The member couple can contribute their experiences for discussion and information-sharing.

Yet another possible dilemma facing leaders is the potential for emotionally attached or ambivalent members to frequently revert to lengthy discussion of their former spouse and life togehter. It must be gently and firmly reinforced that the focus of the group is not analysis of the past marriage. Rather, the group purpose is concerned with how one must accept a single status and function capably in that position in interactions with absent or ex-spouse, children, families of origin, work place, dating partners, and friends. The former task of analysis of past marriages, if needed, is better handled in concurrent therapy. Thus the leader must focus sessions in the here-and-now with emphasis on meeting the present emotional and situational needs of the single person and parent.

SUMMARY

In conclusion, those persons who remain emotionally attached or ambivalent to their ex-spousal partners despite marital dissolution or separation are impeded in their recovery from the divorce consequences. Before this population can initiate the normal restructuring tasks following separation or divorce, they must first emotionally accept the reality of their situation and the consequent changes. This paper is an attempt to help identify persons who are at risk of engaging in continued emotional attachment or ambivalence and how group work may intervene to hasten emotional acceptance and readiness to engage in restructuring of their intrapsychic and interpersonal situations.

NOTE

1. Kitson (1982) reported that 42% of her U.S. sample had separated at least once prior to divorce, while Weiss (1975) similarly suggested that half of all U.S. couples separated at least once during married life.

REFERENCES

Bohannon, P. (1970) Six stages of Divorce. In P. Bohannon (ed.) *Divorce and after*. New York: Doubleday and Co.

Brown, E. (1976a) A model of the divorce Process. *Conciliation Court Review. 14* (2), 1–10.

Brown, E. (1976b) Divorce counselling in treating relationships. In D. Olson (ed.) *Treating relationships*. Iowa: Graphic Publishing Company.

Brown, P., Felton, B., Whiteman, V. & Manela, R. (1980) Attachment and distress following separation. *Journal of Divorce. 3* (4), 303–318.

Cuber, J. & Harroff, P. (1965) *Sex and the significant Americans*. New York: Pelican Books.

Goode, W. (1956) *After divorce*. New York: MacMillan.

Goode, W. (1966) Marital satisfaction and instability. In R. Bendix and S. Lipset (eds.) *Class status and power*. New York: Collier & MacMillan.

Hetherington, E., Cox, M. & Cox, R. (1976) Divorced fathers. *Family Co-ordinator. 25* (4), 417–428.

Kitson, G. (1982) Attachment to spouse in divorce: A scale and its application. *Journal of Marriage and Family. 44* (2), 379–394.

Kressel, K. (1980) Patterns of coping in divorce and some implications for clinical treatment. *Family Relations*. *29* (2), 234–240.

Kressel, K., Jaffee, N., Tuchman, B., Watson, W. & Deutsch, M. (1980) A typology of divorcing couples: Implications for mediation and the divorce process. *Family Process*. *19* (2), 101–116.

Kurdek, L. & Blisk, B. (1983) Dimensions and correlates of mothers' divorce experiences. *Journal of Divorce*. *6* (4), 1–24.

Lang, N. (1981) Social work practice in small social forms: Some unacknowledged entities. Paper presented at Third Annual Symposium on Social Work with Groups. Hartford, Connecticut.

Levinger, G. (1965) Marital cohesiveness and dissolution: An integrative review. *Journal of Marriage and Family*. *27* (1), 19–28.

Marris, P. (1974) *Loss and change*. New York: Pantheon.

Moles, O. & Levinger, G. (1976) In conclusion: Threads in the fabric. *Journal of Social Issues*. *32* (1), 193–207.

Nass, S. (1977) *Crisis intervention*. Iowa: Kendall/Hunt Pub. Company.

Power, R. (in press) Emotional attachment and ambivalence: An indicator for pre-mediation counselling. *Conciliation Court Review*.

Raschke, H. (1977) The role of social participation in post-separation and post-divorce adjustment. *Journal of Divorce*. *1* (1), 129–140.

Spanier, G. & Casto, R. (1979) Adjustment to separation and divorce: A qualitative analysis. In G. Levinger and O.C. Moles (eds.) *Divorce and separation*. New York: Basic Books.

Sprenkle, D. & Storm, C. (1982) Individual treatment in divorce therapy: A critique of an assumption. *Journal of Divorce*. *6* (1/2), 87–97.

Statistics Canada. (1983) *Divorce: Law and the Family in Canada*.

Weiss, R. (1975) *Marital separation*. New York: Basic Books.

Yalom, I. (1975) *The theory and practice of group psychotherapy*. sec. ed. New York: Basic Books.

Zeiss, A., Zeiss, R. & Johnson, S. (1980) Sex differences in initiation of and adjustment to divorce. *Journal of Divorce*. *4* (2), 21–33.

An Evaluation of the "Recovery of Hope" Program

Virginia Moxley
Kenneth Eggeman
Walter R. Schumm

ABSTRACT. The Recovery of Hope program was initiated in 1981 to address the problem of couples entering marriage enrichment events whose distress levels indicated a need for therapy rather than enrichment. An ex post facto evaluation was conducted for this divorce prevention program, surveying 190 spouses who had been involved in the program prior to October 1984. Returns were obtained from 34 wives and 27 husbands on post-test and retrospective pre-test marital satisfaction measures, along with a variety of other items and demographic data. Program completion appeared to assist couples in either improving their relationship or in deciding to divorce, as opposed to continuing with an unsatisfactory marital relationship.

In the early phases of divorce therapy, an important goal is related to the couple's decision to either divorce or to continue working on improving their marriage. Such decisions are complicated and confusing. Kressel and Deutsch (1977) have observed a prevalence of client misdiagnosis of whether the marriage is worth saving, with some clients hoping for the impossible and others giving up too quickly. Turner (1985: 28) cites Janis (1982) who concluded that the divorce oriented person begins to narrow the number of options seen, overlooks long-term implications, ignores information and data normally considered, becomes error prone in

---

Virginia Moxley, PhD, is Associate Dean of the College of Human Ecology, Kansas State University. Kenneth Eggeman, PhD, is Director of Life Directions Programs, Regis College, Denver, Co. Walter R. Schumm, PhD, is Associate Professor, Department of Human Development and Family Studies, Justin Hall, Kansas State University, Manhattan, KS 66506. Work reported here was supported in part by the Kansas Agricultural Experiment Station, contribution number 86-350-J. Requests for reprints should be sent to the third author. Appreciation is expressed to Kristal Bradshaw for her assistance in locating some of the previous research cited in this report.

assessing expected results, and oversimplifies the decision making procedures one would normally utilize. Turner himself (1985: 27) observes that when a person decides for divorce, he or she is often under a very high level of stress and can unknowingly seek premature closure by making the decision in order to escape the anxiety, worry, and anger.

While most professionals would agree upon the important role of professional support for spouses during the process of such decision making, the value orientation of the therapist toward "saving marriages" or conversely, "rescuing victims of bad marriages," can also affect the direction of therapy (Salts, 1985: 16). On occasion one finds certain types of intervention (e.g., excluding one spouse from therapy, Salts, 1985; Whitaker & Miller, 1971: 254) or therapist attitudes (Lazrus, 1981) reflecting a more favorable stance towards divorce. Others, such as Salts (1985: 15), take a more neutral stance, suggesting that "The decision to divorce must be the client's and the therapist should remain as neutral as possible toward the decision regarding the maintenance or dissolution of the marital relationship." However, some therapists, including the staff for Recovery of Hope, take a more positive attitude toward marriage and may try to design a program that has an expressed goal of helping couples avoid divorce and to improve their marriage, while at the same time recognizing that a certain percentage of couples will divorce in any event—and that such an outcome should not always be construed as failure but may represent a measure of the program's success (Framo, 1985).

Although a larger number of reports on the effectiveness of divorce adjustment therapy and mediation are available (Hozman & Froiland, 1976; Goldman & Coane, 1977; Granvold & Welch, 1979; Wallerstein & Kelly, 1977; Elkin, 1977; Bonkowski & Wanner-Westly, 1979; Coche & Goldman, 1979; Hassall & Madar, 1980; Bahr, 1981; Davis, 1983; Huber, 1983; Davidoff & Schiller, 1983), relatively few programs have been reported in which attempts have been made to "save" marriages of couples already seriously considering divorce (Sprenkle & Storm, 1983). We are aware of three programs that have been evaluated among those oriented towards preventing divorce. Hight (1977) reported a 92% success rate for preserving marriages among 25 couples in a program that required that *both* spouses express doubt about the desirability of getting a divorce. Toomin (1972) worked with 18 couples and reported that six (33%) couples reinstated their marriages, while the rest (67%) did divorce. In a study of a program that had dealt with 73 couples, Greene, Lee & Lustig (1973) reported 23% improved marriages, 33% stable but not improved marriages, and 44% divorces.

The following report is an ex post facto evaluation of one such program designed to "save" the marriages of couples that were at the point of seriously considering divorce.

PROGRAM GOALS AND CONTENT

The "Recovery of Hope" program was founded in October 1981 by the late Dr. Sheldon Louthan and professional counselors Floyd and Nelda Coleman at the Family Center of Friends University in Wichita, Kansas. The program was initiated when it continued to be apparent that between 15 and 25 percent of couples attending marriage enrichment events could benefit more from marital therapy than from marital enrichment. Not only was the marriage enrichment experience inappropriate for these troubled couples, but their presence was interfering with the enrichment experience for those with healthier marriages.

Therefore, the Recovery of Hope program was designed and copyrighted to assist couples contemplating divorce in (1) regaining hope that they could avoid divorce and improve their marriage and in (2) linking up with a reputable, appropriate professional counselor who could help each couple decide on the future direction and shape of their relationship. The program was based on several assumptions including (1) despair and marital dissatisfaction lower the amount of effort a husband and wife are willing to expend in renewing their marriage, (2) a renewed sense of hope will increase the effort, including efforts to seek counseling and other remedial assistance, they are willing to expend, and (3) meeting with other couples who had overcome similarly deeply painful problems would tend to reduce discouragement and raise hopes enough to allow couples to make more careful decisions about their relationship. The introductory session is designed to last three hours. Presenting couples who have experienced severe marital problems and have gotten back together after therapy (along with special training) share their experiences, the hurt and hopelessness and reconciliation they experienced in their marriages. Immediately after the presenting couple have shared their presentation, a counselor assists each participating couple with developing a joint contract that outlines a plan for counseling and remedial services. Not all couples who register for

Recovery of Hope decide to enter counseling or sign a contract. Program attrition is shown in Table 1. Since counselors are free to conduct therapy sessions for Recovery of Hope as they wish, subsequent treatments are not identical in content or format, though in most cases, couples have been seen conjointly by one counselor rather than individually or by co-therapists. In essence, the standard practice follows Storm & Sprenkle's (1982) recommendation for conjoint therapy in the early phases of the divorce process.

Presenting couples were trained during the fall of 1981. The first session for participating couples was in February 1982. When Friends University closed the Family Center in the summer of 1982, the program was transferred to the Pastoral Associates group of Wichita, which is an outreach arm of Prairie View, Inc., a private non-profit psychiatric hospital providing outpatient clinical services at four locations. The present director is Stephen K. Wilke, PhD.[1] The program is currently expanding nationwide, with the first satellite program having begun in central Pennsylvania in October 1985.

EVALUATION DESIGN

In the period between February 1982 and September 1984, 196 persons (95 couples and 6 individual spouses) registered to participate in the Recovery of Hope program, which was advertised

TABLE 1

Event	Husbands	Wives
Registered for Recovery of Hope	27 (100%)	34 (100%)
Registered but did not attend first or subsequent sessions	5	7
Registered and did attend first session	22 (81.5%)	27 (79.4%)
Attended first session but did not sign contract	11	10
Attended first session and signed contract	11 (40.8%)	17 (50.0%)
Signed contract but did not complete it	4	7
Signed and completed contract for the Recovery of Hope program	7 (25.9%)	10 (29.4%)

locally by Pastoral Associates, Prairie View, and Friends University. Participants were counseled by 14 different counselors in the sessions couples agreed to in their contracts; however, the largest amount of the counseling was conducted by the Colemans and Dr. Louthan.

Pastoral Associates contracted with the authors to conduct an ex post facto evaluation of the effectiveness of the program in the summer of 1984 and granted permission for publication of the results. No attempt was made to contact the individual spouses; however, of the 95 couples, 91 couples and four spouses were located through their respective counselors and local telephone directories (the other four spouses could not be located). Surveys were mailed to each participant in November 1984. Follow-up surveys were sent in January 1985 to individuals who had not responded to the first survey. Responses were received from both spouses from 18 of the 91 couples (20%) and from 16 other wives and 9 husbands for a partial to complete response rate from 43 of the 95 couples (45%). Sprenkle & Storm (1983) and Salts & Zongker (1983) have observed that time is important for assessing the effectiveness of divorce or reconciliation therapy, with the former recommending a follow-up interval of at least six months to assess the permanence of reported changes associated with therapy. In this evaluation, the spouses completed their surveys between five and 36 months after initiating the program with an average time of 17.6 (SD = 9.3) months for husbands and 18.6 (SD = 9.9) months for wives.[2]

RESPONDENT CHARACTERISTICS

Husbands' ages ranged from 22 to 59 years (M = 38.1, SD = 9.23), and wives' from 23 to 59 (M = 36.1, SD = 9.2). Duration of marriage ranged from 3 to 32 years for husbands (M = 14.2, SD = 8.65) and 2 to 34 years for wives (M = 13.8, SD = 9.12).[3] Nine of the husbands and seven of the wives had a high school education or less, while seven husbands and eleven wives had college degrees. Eleven of the husbands and fifteen wives reported family incomes of less than $20,000 per year while 13 husbands and 16 wives reported incomes of $20,000 or more.

Of 27 husbands who responded, 14 were married, 2 had separated, and 11 had divorced since the program; of the 34 wives who responded, 20 were married, one had separated, and 13 had divorced. Most of the husbands had not had any premarital counseling (61.5%), while another 3.8% had had only very brief premarital counseling. Likewise, 57.6% of the wives had had no premarital counseling and another 9.1% had had only very brief premarital counseling. In terms of church attendance, 57.6% of the wives and 69.3% of the husbands reported attending church at least once a month with their spouses at the time they registered for the Recovery of Hope program. Most of the husbands (77.8%) and wives (78.8%) had been married only once when they registered for Recovery of Hope. All others, with the exception of two wives in their third marriage, had only been married twice.

MEASUREMENT

The Kansas Marital Satisfaction Scale was used to assess current marital satisfaction for those still married and to assess marital satisfaction at the time of participation in the Recovery of Hope program, as retrospectively reported by the subjects. Divorced subjects did not report their current marital satisfaction. Previous research reports summarized in Schumm, Anderson, Benigas, McCutchen, Griffin, Morris, & Race (1985) have provided evidence for the high internal consistency reliability and test-retest reliability of the KMS scale, while that summary provided some evidence for criterion-related validity since the scale discriminated between intact and separated couples. A more recent report (Schumm, Paff-Bergen, Hatch, Obiorah, Copeland, Meens, & Bugaighis, in press) has provided evidence for the concurrent validity of the KMS scale with Spanier's (1976) Dyadic Adjustment Scale and Norton's (1983) Quality Marriage Index. Other studies have provided some evidence for the construct validity of the KMS scale (Anderson, Russell, & Schumm, 1983; Schumm & Bugaighis, in press; Copeland, Bugaighis, & Schumm, 1984; Grover, Russell, Schumm, & Paff-Bergen, 1985; Schumm, Jurich, Bollman, & Bugaighis, 1985; Eggeman, Moxley, & Schumm, 1985; Barnes, Schumm, Jurich, & Bollman, 1984; Bugaighis, Schumm, Jurich, & Bollman, 1985).

Cronbach (1951) *alpha* estimates of internal consistency reliability were .86 for 26 husbands and .88 for 33 wives at "pre-program" and .92 for 15 husbands and .98 for 19 wives at the present time. For all but the "pre-program" wives, the relative means for the items in the KMS scale paralleled previous research, with least satisfaction being reported for relationship with spouse and the greatest satisfaction being reported for satisfaction with partner as a spouse. Mean scores on the KMS scale were low, as might be expected from the population involved, M = 7.96 (SD = 4.49) for "pre-program" husbands; M = 10.47 (SD = 6.24) for husbands at present; M = 6.67 (SD = 4.07) for "pre-program" wives; and M = 12.74 (SD = 6.14) for wives at present. Those scores compare favorably to the mean score, M = 10.13 (SD = 5.33), obtained for separated wives in the Schumm, Anderson et al. (1985) study.

Single items were used to assess how often (five categories from almost never to almost always) subjects had agreed on common goals and values for their marriage (Q1), communicated effectively about their relationship and individual needs (Q2), tried new ways of dealing with problems and compromising to settle disagreements (Q3), expressed appreciation and affection for one another (Q4), agreed upon one another's roles and responsibilities (Q5), shared household responsibilites fairly (Q6), achieved sexual satisfaction (Q7), satisfactorily managed the family income (Q8), consulted each other on important issues in order to make wise and acceptable decisions (Q9), believed they were good parents (Q10), and were committed to improving their relationship (Q11). As with the KMS scale, each of the eleven items was asked with respect to the present time and with respect to the time when the subject had begun to participate in Recovery of Hope.

ANALYSIS

Two statistical designs were used to evaluate the Recovery of Hope program. One-way analyses of variance were used to predict a variety of demographic variables from the independent variable of marital status for which subjects were classified as (1) divorced, (2) in intact but unimproved marriages, and (3) in intact, improved marriages. Repeated measures analyses of variance were used to compare retrospective "pre-program" scores with current scores, using between subjects factors of program completion status and length of marriage. Categories of program completion status were (1) registered, but did not attend the introductory session, (2) attended the introductory session but did not sign Recovery of Hope contract, (3) signed, but did not complete the contract, and (4) completed the contract. To reduce the number of cells involved with the smaller number of subjects, the program completion status codes were recorded into two levels—either program completed (4 recoded to 2) or program not completed (1, 2, and 3 recoded to 1). It was hypothesized that program completion would be associated with apparent gains from "pre-program" to current marital satisfaction scores and possibly with several of the single items (Q1 through Q11), particularly those items dealing with interpersonal interaction, negotiation, communication (as opposed to financial management, being good parents, and responsibilities) which were probably more valued outcomes by most of the Recovery of Hope staff and the counselors. Categories of length of marriage were recoded to (1) married ten years or less and (2) married 11 years or more. It was hypothesized that having been married for a longer time would be predictive of greater improvement because of the increased investment in the relationship (Brown & Manela, 1977; Lee, 1979).

$SPSS^x$ routines (SPSS, Inc., 1983) were used to perform all analyses; the repeated measures analyses were patterned after the procedures discussed in Schumm, Bugaighis, & Jurich (1985) and elsewhere (O'Brien & Kaiser, 1985). Because no current marital satisfaction scores were available for divorced individuals, each repeated measures analysis was run two ways—first, only with subjects who did not divorce and secondly, with all subjects, substituting "pre-program" scores for the missing current scores of the divorced subjects.

RESULTS

One-way analyses of variance for age, education, duration of marriage, income, number of previous marriages, size of community, prior premarital counseling, and percentage of fees paid by subject for the program all proved to be nonsignificant. The only significant result was that the percentages[4] of husband and wives in each of the three categories of the independent variable varied in terms of having seen a professional counselor as part of the Recovery of Hope program. For husbands, 91% (10 of 11) of those who divorced saw a counselor; 38% (3 of 8) of those whose marriage stayed intact but no happier saw a counselor; and 100% of those seven husbands whose marriage improved saw a counselor.

The difference was significant by $F(2, 23) = 7.56$ ($p = .003$). For wives, $F(2, 30) = 4.09$ ($p = .027$) with 92% (12 of 13) of divorced wives, 40% (2 of 5) of those with intact but unimproved marriages and 87% (13 of 15) of wives with improved marriages having seen a counselor. Thus, it would appear that seeing a counselor served as a catalyst for marital change, either enabling it to succeed or confirming its lack of potential for permanence (Table 2).

Detailed results are presented for marital satisfaction as the dependent variable (Tables 3 through 6), but results are abbreviated for the remaining items in order to conserve space (Tables 7 and 8). For husbands, program completion appeared to facilitate positive changes in marital satisfaction, agreement on goals (Q1), effective communication (Q2), conflict resolution (Q3), expression of appreciation (Q4), decision-making (Q9), and commitment (Q11). For husbands married over 10 years who completed the program, positive change also occurred on the variables of agreement upon roles (Q5) and achievement of sexual satisfaction (Q7). Some changes occurred in marital satisfaction and items Q1, Q2, Q3, Q4, Q5, and Q11 regardless of program completion, as shown by significant results for the "Time" factor by itself, independent of program completion or duration of marriage factors.

For wives, the results are not so clear cut. On all variables except agreement upon goals (Q1), achievement of sexual satisfaction (Q7), and commitment (Q11), wives appeared to improve regardless of program completion. Program completion appeared to facilitate change only for marital satisfaction and agreement on roles (Q5). Wives married over 10 years seemed to respond more positively to Recovery of Hope program completion than wives married ten years or less in terms of the variables of expression of appreciation (Q4), agreement on roles (Q5), income management (Q8), confidence in parenting (Q10), and commitment (Q11).

For both husbands and wives, the inclusion of substituted data for divorced spouses did not appear to make much difference for the "time" effect, but it did seem to yield stronger results for the "time by program completion" effect. In contrast, results for the "duration of marriage by program completion by time" effect were stronger for the analyses that did not include the scores for the couples divorced at the current time. However, in the majority of cases, if an effect was significant by one technique, it was also significant by the other technique.

TABLE 2

Percentage of Husbands and Wives in Each Present Marital Status Who Saw a Counselor

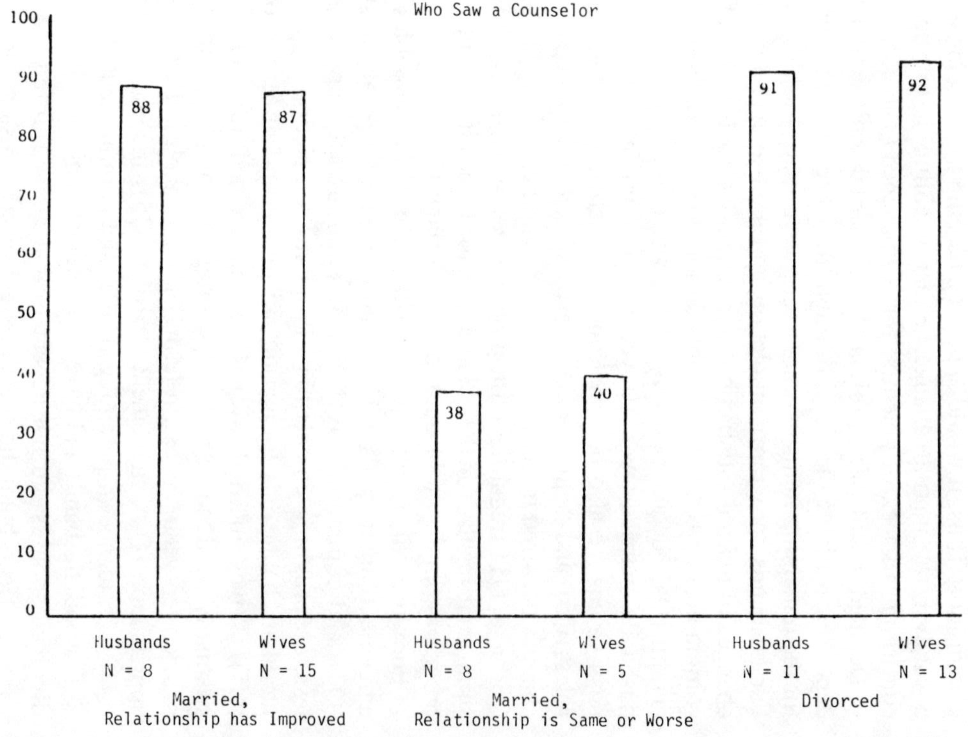

Participants were also invited to comment on the program in an open-ended question at the end of the survey questionnaire. Some comments were negative, with the content of the first session drawing most of the criticism. One husband felt that couples were not adequately warned in the first session about the likelihood of suppressed anger arising and hurting feelings. One wife said that the first session seemed "too canned," almost humiliating for the presenting couples. Another spouse said that the appeal to emotionalism was not appropriate for people going through life crises. Negative comments on the overall program included,

> "The program really isn't anything, just a two-hour shot and going off to see a counselor."

> "It just made us feel guilty when we failed and others were succeeding."

For other participants, the program was seen as good, but either too

TABLE 3

Source	SS	df	MS	F	p
Between Subjects[a]					
Program Completion (A)	87.55	1	87.55	3.75	.082
Duration of Marriage (B)	4.96	1	4.96	0.21	.655
A x B	57.38	1	57.38	2.46	.148
Error	233.63	10	23.36		
Within Subjects					
"Time" (C)	142.36	1	142.36	45.49	.000
A x C	154.41	1	154.41	49.35	.000
B x C	11.00	1	11.00	3.52	.090
A x B x C	19.41	1	19.41	6.20	.032
Error	31.29	10	3.13		

[a] The Bartlett test for homogeneity of covariance matrices was not significant (i.e., the cells associated with the between subjects factors have similar covariance structures).

TABLE 4

Source	SS	df	MS	F	p
Between Subjects					
Program Completion (A)	59.41	1	59.41	1.64	.214
Duration of Marriage (B)	3.74	1	3.74	0.10	.751
A x B	95.77	1	95.77	2.65	.119
Error	760.10	21	36.20		
Within Subjects					
"Time" (C)	119.70	1	119.70	27.10	.000
A x C	126.10	1	126.10	28.54	.000
B x C	1.14	1	1.14	0.26	.617
A x B x C	2.90	1	2.90	0.66	.427
Error	92.77	21	4.42		

[a] The Bartlett test for homogeneity of covariance matrices was significant, Box's M = 24.12, $F(6,257) = 2.93$ ($p = .009$) and $X^2(6) = 18.17$ ($p = .006$). Therefore, results must be interpreted cautiously.

late or ineffective at enlisting their spouse's cooperation. Comments included:

> "It was a good program, but my marriage was too far gone."
>
> "I wish we'd have known about it and realized we needed it a long time ago."
>
> "Recovery of Hope and two other programs have not helped in getting our marriage back together. I cannot find fault with any of the programs."
>
> "I think the program is very good for the most part. I only wish we had participated."
>
> "We are still having great marital problems but my spouse will not deal with them."
>
> "I believe if my spouse was open minded and willing to work out our problems that we might still be married."

> "I thought we had a chance to save our marriage but my spouse refused to go through the program. I never knew why. It appeared as though the program could have helped us."

Some participants felt the program was successful in helping them make a wise decision to divorce—"Recovery of Hope helped me see how hopeless recovery for our marriage was." "My ex-wife and I are still very good friends."

Positive comments include:

> "One point of major help was just to see how others' problems were more extreme than ours and they had worked them out."
>
> "The program helped us to continue working on our problems."
>
> "It definitely did give me new hope."
>
> "We are expecting our first child soon and are extremely happy. Success!"

TABLE 5

Source	SS	df	MS	F	p
Between Subjects					
Program Completion (A)	22.04	1	22.04	0.78	.393
Duration of Marriage (B)	11.44	1	11.44	0.40	.535
A x B	4.43	1	4.43	0.16	.699
Error	396.64	14	28.33		
Within Subjects					
"Time" (C)	420.56	1	420.56	35.67	.000
A x C	41.60	1	41.60	3.53	.081
B x C	12.02	1	12.02	1.02	.330
A x B x C	28.72	1	28.72	2.44	.141
Error	165.07	14	11.79		

[a] The Bartlett test for homogeneity of covariance matrices was not significant.

"I have recommended your program to several people who are having marriage problems."

"The sessions were valuable in most every aspect."

DISCUSSION

Recovery of Hope worked for some subjects; it did not seem to work for others. Although six husbands and eight wives indicated in the comment section of the survey that the program had a positive effect on their marriages, two husbands and three wives indicated that the program had a negative effect; in addition, five husbands and four wives indicated that the program was good, but that either they didn't fully participate or that it was too late to do any good for their marriage. From these comments, it appears that Recovery of Hope probably works most effectively at linking couples up with a professional counselor. This overcomes resistance to "therapy" by allowing couples to enter via a more optimistic sounding "program," which provides some motivation during the initial session for subsequent counseling. For those who expect the initial session

TABLE 6

Source	SS	df	MS	F	p
Between Subjects					
Program Completion (A)	19.95	1	19.95	0.56	.467
Duration of Marriage (B)	0.70	1	0.70	0.02	.891
A x B	6.47	1	6.47	0.18	.678
Error	987.73	27	36.58		
Within Subjects					
"Time" (C)	277.91	1	277.91	22.11	.000
A x C	69.48	1	69.48	5.53	.026
B x C	0.57	1	0.57	0.05	.832
A x B x C	7.03	1	7.03	0.56	.461
Error	339.44	27	12.57		

[a] The Bartlett test for homogeneity of covariance matrices was not significant.

TABLE 7

Variable	Mean Scores: "Pre-Test" Did Not Complete Program Younger	"Pre-Test" Did Not Complete Program Older	"Pre-Test" Did Complete Program Younger	"Pre-Test" Did Complete Program Older	"Post-Test" Did Not Complete Program Younger	"Post-Test" Did Not Complete Program Older	"Post-Test" Did Complete Program Younger	"Post-Test" Did Complete Program Older	Results: "Time"	A x C	A x B x C	A x B x C Bartlett
KMS	4.75[a]	9.33	8.50	3.00	5.00	8.67	15.5	16.5	.000	.000	.032	
	5.63	10.08	8.50	4.67	5.75	9.75	15.5	13.67	.000	.000	.427	
Q1	1.67	3.00	3.50	1.50	2.33	2.83	4.50	4.00	.007	.029	.074	
	2.14	3.17	3.50	2.67	2.43	3.08	4.50	4.33	.002	.008	.227	
Q2	1.00	2.33	3.00	2.00	1.33	2.00	4.00	4.00	.005	.005	.072	(*)
	1.57	2.33	3.00	2.67	1.71	2.17	4.00	4.00	.001	.001	.310	
Q3	1.67	2.83	3.50	1.50	1.67	2.50	4.50	4.00	.011	.004	.096	
	1.57	2.55	3.50	2.33	1.57	2.36	4.50	4.00	.004	.001	.279	
Q4	1.67	3.00	3.00	1.00	2.33	2.83	4.50	4.00	.000	.001	.019	(*)
	2.14	2.75	3.00	1.67	2.43	2.67	4.50	3.67	.000	.000	.265	(*)
Q5	1.67	2.80	3.00	2.00	2.33	2.60	3.00	4.00	.016	.097	.008	
	1.71	2.50	3.00	2.67	2.00	2.40	3.00	4.00	.030	.093	.016	
Q6	2.67	3.60	2.50	3.50	2.67	3.40	3.00	3.50	.774	.507	.774	(*)
	2.43	3.40	2.50	3.33	2.43	3.30	3.00	3.33	.490	.305	.490	(*)
Q7	3.67	2.00	4.50	2.50	3.67	1.67	4.00	4.00	.313	.061	.005	(*)
	3.14	2.50	4.50	2.33	3.14	2.33	4.00	3.33	.436	.171	.002	
Q8	2.33	3.67	4.50	4.50	2.67	3.83	4.50	4.00	.999	.117	.578	
	1.86	3.25	4.50	4.00	2.00	3.33	4.50	3.67	.769	.135	.455	
Q9	3.00	4.00	3.50	3.50	2.67	3.50	4.50	4.50	.279	.021	.873	
	2.29	3.64	3.50	4.00	2.14	3.36	4.50	4.67	.072	.005	.760	
Q10	3.67	4.50	4.00	3.50	4.00	4.50	4.00	4.00	.161	.766	.161	(*)
	3.83	4.25	4.00	4.00	4.00	4.25	4.00	4.33	.186	.652	.186	
Q11	3.00	3.80	3.50	1.50	2.67	3.40	4.50	5.00	.040	.009	.134	
	3.43	3.91	3.50	2.67	3.29	3.73	4.50	5.00	.012	.003	.223	

(*) indicates that Bartlett test either could not be performed or that it was significant.

[a] For each variable, the top row represents data for intact couples only. The bottom row represents results for intact and divorced spouses, with data substitution for divorced spouses for the current scores.

TABLE 8

	Mean Scores								Results		
	"Pre-Test"				"Post-Test"						
	Did Not Complete Program		Did Complete Program		Did Not Complete Program		Did Complete Program		"Time"	A x C	A x B x C
	Younger	Older	Younger	Older	Younger	Older	Younger	Older			
KMS	5.14[a]	6.25	5.67	4.50	10.71	10.50	12.00	17.00	.000	.081	.141
	6.77	6.33	5.67	5.17	9.77	8.22	12.00	13.50	.000	.026	.461
Q1	2.57	3.50	3.67	2.75	3.14	3.75	3.33	4.25	.132	.785	.105
	2.67	3.33	3.67	2.83	3.00	3.44	3.33	3.83	.196	.793	.074
Q2	1.71	2.00	1.33	2.00	2.57	3.25	2.67	3.75	.000	.385	.983
	1.92	1.78	1.33	2.00	2.42	2.33	2.67	3.17	.000	.099	.795
Q3	1.86	2.50	2.00	1.50	3.14	3.50	3.33	4.50	.000	.151	.170
	1.75	2.22	2.00	1.67	2.50	2.67	3.33	3.67	.000	.062	.384
Q4	1.57	3.25	2.67	1.75	2.71	3.50	3.00	3.50	.004	.511	.041
	2.17	2.56	2.67	2.00	2.83	2.67	3.00	3.17	.007	.366	.088
Q5	1.71	3.50	2.33	2.50	2.57	3.25	3.00	4.00	.000	.022	.006
	2.50	2.78	2.33	2.17	3.00	2.67	3.00	3.17	.001	.024	.087
Q6	1.57	3.00	2.00	2.25	2.43	3.50	2.67	3.75	.009	.499	.325
	1.67	2.44	2.00	2.00	2.17	2.67	2.67	3.00	.007	.260	.463
Q7	2.57	2.50	4.00	2.75	3.43	2.25	3.67	3.75	.380	.967	.104
	3.50	2.44	4.00	2.67	4.00	2.33	3.67	3.33	.441	.952	.093 (*)
Q8	3.29	4.50	3.33	3.25	3.86	4.50	3.33	4.50	.006	.244	.006
	3.00	3.44	3.33	3.33	3.33	3.44	3.33	4.17	.015	.274	.015
Q9	2.71	4.50	2.67	3.25	3.71	4.50	3.00	4.50	.018	.556	.068
	2.67	3.78	2.67	3.00	3.25	3.78	3.00	3.83	.019	.413	.135
Q10	3.60	4.25	5.00	3.50	4.20	4.50	4.50	4.50	.024	.512	.004
	4.00	4.11	5.00	3.67	4.27	4.22	4.50	4.33	.204	.611	.004
Q11	3.57	3.67	4.67	3.00	3.71	3.67	3.67	5.00	.347	.478	.019 (*)
	3.92	3.88	4.67	3.67	4.00	3.88	3.67	5.00	.604	.755	.005 (*)

(*) indicates that Bartlett test either could not be performed or that it was significant.

[a] For each variable, the top row represents data for intact couples only. The bottom row represents results for intact and divorced spouses, with data substitution for divorced spouses for the current scores.

to do anything else therapeutic, the program may fail. Once into counseling, the experience seemed to create a climate for change for many couples, helping them to clarify for themselves the direction they wanted their relationship to take as opposed to allowing things to drag on without change. Those couples who saw a counselor generally opted for divorce or improving their relationship, while those who didn't see a counselor generally continued in an unsatisfactory relationship. Counselors may not have saved marriages as much as helped couples work through what they wanted to do with their marriage, to work harder at saving it or to terminate it rather than letting things drag on in an inconclusive condition. This "splitting effect" by itself suggests that Recovery of Hope is serving the useful function of helping couples clarify their personal and relationship goals, which is a standard objective of the early phases of divorce therapy (Turner, 1985; Salts, 1985; Hight, 1977; Toomim, 1972).

In spite of the lack of control over therapist service delivery (the possible heterogeneity of treatment effects), the percentage of marriages "saved" versus those ending in divorce or continuing in an unsatisfactory manner appears to be comparable to other programs similar to Recovery of Hope (Toomim, 1972; Greene, Lee, & Lustig, 1973). Recovery of Hope, like other programs, cannot be expected to prevent all divorces, but it may prevent some. Prevention of unnecessary divorce and improved marital satisfaction is the goal of the program. Some couples use the program to help themselves recognize the inevitability of divorce and to act upon their decision. Of course, some couples who did not divorce felt that their relationship quality had not improved or had deteriorated even though marital stability was preserved; however, those couples were most likely to be the ones who did *not* participate fully in the Recovery of Hope program.

In terms of the repeated measures analyses, it appears that on five variables (KMS scale, Q2, Q3, Q4, and Q5) husbands and wives improved over time, regardless of program completion and that on five others either the husband (Q1, Q11) or the wife (Q6, Q8, Q9) improved. That result could reflect many things besides a valid treatment effect—subjects desiring to "thank" the program, genuine improvement associated with treatment effects from agencies outside the Recovery of Hope program, etc. The only variables for which the program appeared to help *both* husbands and wives were marital satisfaction and agreement upon roles (Q5), with improvement on the latter occurring mostly for those couples who had been married longer. While program completion also appeared helpful for husbands in terms of agreement on goals (Q1), effective communication (Q2), conflict resolution (Q3), expression of appreciation (Q4), decision-making (Q9), and commitment (Q11), it was not helpful for wives in terms of anything other than marital satisfaction or agreement upon roles (Q5), with the exception that wives married over 10 years appeared to improve in terms of income management (Q8), parenting (Q10) and commitment (Q11).

In summary, Recovery of Hope appeared to benefit husbands more than wives, although both spouses appeared to improve as a result of program completion in terms of marital satisfaction, which was perhaps the most valid measure used. The program may have helped couples a bit more when they had more invested in preserving their marriage. In conclusion, it appears that couples who complete their contracts and counseling experience are either helped to improve their relationship or to terminate it, although husbands and those spouses who are more invested in their relationship may benefit more in some aspects.

Our evaluation of the Recovery of Hope program has very obvious limitations in terms of the standards proposed by Sprenkle & Storm (1983). In particular, no control group was available for this after-the-fact evaluation; the best we could do was to investigate the ''time'' effect to see if improvement was associated with time or memory effects by themselves independent of treatment effects—and some evidence for such was found. The sample size was less than ideal, but probably not too different than most other studies. The sample was not random and the response rate from the total population of participants was only 45% at best. The follow-up was probably reasonable but the time was not standard because the treatments were not standard and the date of termination of treatment was not obtained during the survey. The client variable of duration of marriage was considered but it was not possible to consider many others in the repeated measures design because of the small sample, although other variables were considered in the one-way analyses of variance. As noted previously, treatments were not standardized; however, the nature of the program itself, as a way of referring couples to therapy does not lend itself to standardized treatment within a realistic community environment. (It's unlikely that the best therapy for each of the referrals would be identical; giving every couple the same treatment would probably be detrimental to some of them.) The outcome criteria were brief self-report measures, less than ideal in some respects, but realistic within the constraints of the project and the use of survey data. The use of the Kansas Marital Satisfaction Scale may be seen as less desirable than a better known instrument such as the Dyadic Adjustment Scale, but its brevity relative to the DAS spoke for its feasibility. Given the initial conditions of the evaluation design—conduct an ex post facto analysis of the program using only survey data in a relatively brief instrument—we think our design and analysis are quite realistic and that our results reflect what may be expected from similar community-based, divorce prevention programs.

NOTES

1. Dr. Wilke may be contacted at National Recovery of Hope, 337 North Waco, Wichita, Kansas 67202 for further information on the program.

2. Time in months since the initiation of the program was *not* significantly correlated with retrospective pre-program or present marital satisfaction for either husbands or wives. The largest correlations, however, were $r = .25$ (p = .15, N = 19) for wives' time versus present marital satisfaction and $r = -.20$ (p = .13, N = 33) for wives' time versus pre-program marital satisfaction. Those correlations, while not significant because of the small N, do suggest that present marital satisfaction may have been either improving with time since program initiation or may have been exaggerated in a "halo"-type effect. The negative correlation may also suggest a "sour grapes" effect, in that subjects may have felt it important to report especially *low* satisfaction prior to the program, either as a way of reconciling themselves to their divorce or highlighting the effectiveness of the program. While our comments are extremely speculative at this point, we think future researchers would do well to investigate such phenomena, which could well have a bearing on the interpretation of results.

3. That is, duration of marriage to spouse to whom married at the time of Recovery of Hope.

4. Since seeing a counselor was a dichotomous variable (0 = no; 1 = yes), mean scores directly reflect percentages; for example, a mean score of .40 reflects 40% of subjects in that category having seen a counselor.

REFERENCES

Anderson, S. A., Russell, C. S., & Schumm, W. R. (1983). Perceived marital quality and family life-cycle categories: a further analysis. *Journal of Marriage and the Family*, 45, 127–139.

Bahr, S. J. Mediation is the answer (1981). *Family Advocate*, 3(4), 32–35.

Barnes, H. L., Schumm, W. R., Jurich, A. P., & Bollman, S. R. (1984). Marital satisfaction: positive regard versus communication as explanatory variables. *Journal of Social Psychology*, 123, 71–78.

Bonkowski, S. E., & Wanner-Westly, B. (1979). The divorce group: a new treatment modality. *Social Casework*, 60, 552–557.

Bugaighis, M. A., Schumm, W. R., Jurich, A. P., & Bollman, S. R. (1985). Factors associated with thought of marital separation. *Journal of Divorce*, 9(2), 49–59.

Coche, J., & Goldman, J. (1979). Brief group psychotherapy for women after divorce: planning a focused experience. *Journal of Divorce*, 3(2), 153–160.

Copland, J. M., Bugaighis, M. A., & Schumm, W. R. (1984). Relationship characteristics of couples married thirty years or more. *Journal of Alternative Lifestyles*, 7, 107–114.

Cronbach, L. J. (1951). Coefficient alpha and the internal structure of tests. *Psychometrika*, 16, 297–334.

Davidoff, I. F., & Schiller, M. S. (1983). The divorce workshop as crisis intervention: a practical model. *Journal of Divorce*, 6(4), 37–53.

Davis, G. (1983). Mediation in divorce: a theoretical perspective. *Journal of Social Welfare Law*, 131–140.

Eggeman, L., Moxley, V., & Schumm, W. R. (1985). Assessing spouses' perceptions of Gottman's temporal form in marital conflict. *Psychological Reports*, 57, 171–181.

Elkin, M. (1977). Postdivorce counseling in a conciliation court. *Journal of Divorce*, 1(1), 55–65.

Framo, J. L. (1985). Breaking the ties that bind. *Family Therapy Networker*, 9(5), 51–56.

Goldman, J., & Coane, J. (1977). Family therapy after the divorce: developing a strategy. *Family Process*, 16, 357–362.

Granvold, D. K., & Welch, G. J. (1979). Structured, short-term group treatment of postdivorce adjustment. *International Journal of Group Psychotherapy*, 24, 347–358.

Greene, B. L., Lee, R. R., & Lustig, N. (1973). Transient structured distance as a manuever in marital therapy. *Family Coordinator*, 20, 15–22.

Grover, K. J., Russell, C. S., Schumm, W. R., & Paff-Bergen, L. A. (1985). Mate selection processes and marital satisfaction. *Family Relations*, 34, 383–386.

Hassall, E., & Madar, D. (1980). Crisis group therapy with the separated and divorced. *Family Relations*, 29, 591–597.

Hight, E. S. (1977). A contractual, working separation: a step between resumption and/or divorce. *Journal of Divorce*, 1(1), 21–30.

Hozman, T. L., & Froiland, D. J. (1976). Families in divorce: a proposed model for counseling the children. *The Family Coordinator*, 25, 271–276.

Huber, C. H. (1983). Divorce mediation: an opportunity for adlerian counselors. *Individual Psychology*, 39, 125–132.

Janis, I. L. (1982). Decisionmaking under stress. In L. Goldberger & S. Breznitz (Eds.), *Handbook of stress, theoretical and clinical aspects*. New York: Free Press.

Kressel, L., & Deutsch, M. (1977). Divorce therapy: an in-depth survey of therapists' views. *Family Process*, 16, 413–443.

Lazrus, A. A. (1981). Divorce counseling or marriage therapy? A therapeutic option. *Journal of Marital and Family Therapy*, 7(1), 15–22.

Norton, R. (1983). Measuring marital quality: a critical look at the dependent variable. *Journal of Marriage and the Family*, 45, 141–151.

O'Brien, R. G., & Kaiser, M. K. (1985). MANOVA method for analyzing repeated measures designs: an extensive primer. *Psychological Bulletin*, 97, 316–333.

Salts, C. J. (1985). Divorce stage theory and therapy: therapeutic implications throughout the divorcing process. *Journal of Psychotherapy and the Family*, 1(3), 13–23.

Salts, C. J., & Zongker, C. E. (1983). Effects of divorce counseling groups on adjustment and self concept. *Journal of Divorce*, 6(4), 55–67.

Schumm, W. R., Anderson, S. A., Benigas, J. E., McCutchen, M. B., Griffin, C. L., Morris, J. E., & Race, G. S. (1985). Criterion-related validity of the Kansas Marital Satisfaction Scale. *Psychological Reports*, 56, 719–722.

Schumm, W. R., & Bugaighis, M. A. Marital quality over the marital career: alternative explanations. *Journal of Marriage and the Family*, in press.

Schumm, W. R., Bugaighis, M. A., & Jurich, A. P. (1985). Using repeated measures designs in program evaluation of family therapy. *Journal of Marital and Family Therapy*, 11, 87–95.

Schumm, W. R., Jurich, A. P., Bollman, S. R., & Bugaighis, M. A. (1985). His and her marriage revisited. *Journal of Family Issues*, 6, 221–227.

Schumm, W. R., Paff-Bergen, L. A., Hatch, R. C., Obiorah, F. C., Copeland, J. M., Meens, L. F., & Bugaighis, M. A. Concurrent and discriminant validity of the Kansas Marital Satisfaction Scale. *Journal of Marriage and the Family*, in press.

Spanier, G. B. (1976). Measuring dyadic adjustment: new scales for assessing the quality of marriage and other dyads. *Journal of Marriage and the Family*, 38, 15–28.

Sprenkle, D. H., & Storm, C. L. (1983). Divorce therapy outcome research: a substantive and methodological review. *Journal of Marital and Family Therapy*, 9, 239–258.

SPSS, Inc. (1983). *SPSS^x user's guide*. New York: McGraw-Hill.

Storm, C. L., & Sprenkle, D. H. (1982). Individaul treatment in divorce therapy: a critique of an assumption. *Journal of Divorce*, 6, 87–97.

Toomim, M. K. (1972). Structured separation with counseling: a therapeutic approach for couples in conflict. *Family Process*, 11, 299–310.

Turner, N. W. (1985). Divorce: dynamics of decision therapy. *Journal of Psychotherapy and the Family*, 1(3), 27–38.

Wallerstein, J. S., & Kelly, J. B. (1977). Divorce counseling: a community service for families in the midst of divorce. *American Journal of Orthopsychiatry*, 47(1), 4–22.

Whitaker, C. A., & Miller, M. S. (1971). Evaluation of "psychiatric" help when divorce impends. In J. Haley (Ed.), *Changing families: a family therapy reader*. New York: Grune & Stratton, 1971.